AF760059

Home Care for Ageing Populations

Home Care for Ageing Populations

A Comparative Analysis of Domiciliary Care in Denmark, the United States and Germany

---

Martha Doyle
Trinity College Dublin, Ireland

and

Virpi Timonen
Trinity College Dublin, Ireland

Edward Elgar
Cheltenham, UK • Northampton, MA, USA

© Martha Doyle and Virpi Timonen 2007

All rights reserved. No part of this publication may be reproduced, stored in a retrieval system or transmitted in any form or by any means, electronic, mechanical or photocopying, recording, or otherwise without the prior permission of the publisher.

Published by
Edward Elgar Publishing Limited
Glensanda House
Montpellier Parade
Cheltenham
Glos GL50 1UA
UK

Edward Elgar Publishing, Inc.
William Pratt House
9 Dewey Court
Northampton
Massachusetts 01060
USA

A catalogue record for this book
is available from the British Library

Library of Congress Cataloguing in Publication Data

Doyle, Martha.
Home care for ageing populations : a comparative analysis of domiciliary care in Denmark, the United States and Germany / by Martha Doyle and Virpi Timonen.
p. cm.
Includes bibliographical references and index.
1. Older people—Home care—Denmark. 2. Older people—Home care—Germany. 3. Older people—Home care—United States. 4. Home care services—Denmark. 5. Home care services—Germany. 6. Home care services—United States. I. Timonen, Virpi. II. Title.
HV1481.D42D68 2007
362.6'3—dc22

2007029876

ISBN 978 1 84720 494 3

Printed and bound in Great Britain by MPG Books Ltd, Bodmin, Cornwall

Contents

Figures

Tables

Notes on Authors

Martha Doyle, MSc (Dublin) is a Research Fellow in the Social Policy and Ageing Research Centre at Trinity College Dublin, Ireland. Virpi Timonen, DPhil (Oxon.) is the Director of the Social Policy and Ageing Research Centre at Trinity College Dublin, Ireland (www.sparc.tcd.ie). The Centre was established in 2005 with a view to producing and disseminating policy-relevant research in the area of ageing.

Acknowledgements

As always, the authors alone are responsible for the contents of this book. We wish to thank the following individuals and institutions for their assistance: Trinity College Dublin Start-up Fund for financing the fieldwork expenses; the Danish Trade Union of Public Employees (FOA) in Copenhagen, the Public Authority in San Francisco and Caritas in Berlin for arranging and coordinating the observation exercises; Margret Steinthorsdottir for translation of Danish documents; the Ministry of Health, Bonn, for the provision of useful contact information; Josephine Doyle for her help in proofreading earlier drafts of the manuscript; Dr Mary Jane Krebbs and Paul Krebbs, for their hospitality and provision of accommodation in New York; Atlantic Philanthropies for supporting the work of the Social Policy and Ageing Research Centre; the Board of the Centre, and in particular Professor Robbie Gilligan, for their support of our work; Ana Diaz who produced the figures in Chapters 2 and 3; Catherine Elgar at Edward Elgar Publishing; Maria Pierce and Margaret Pegh (Edward Elgar Publishing) for their invaluable and thorough proofreading of the final manuscript and David Givens in The Liffey Press for production of the camera ready copy of the manuscript. Finally, a heartfelt thanks to all the individuals in Copenhagen, San Francisco, New York, Berlin and Bonn who generously gave their time to be interviewed. This research would not have been possible without their assistance and cooperation.

1. Introduction: Exploring the Complex Worlds of Domiciliary Care

The umbrella term 'long-term care' for older people encompasses a wide spectrum of services in both community and institutional settings. Care in the community setting can be subdivided into informal and formal care: whereas the former is carried out by family members, neighbours and friends who in most cases are not paid for this work, the latter is carried out by paid workers with varying types and levels of training and qualifications. Formal community care straddles a variety of community-based services such as day centres, meal services, respite care and community nursing services as well as care services provided in the older person's own home such as help with domestic chores, personal care and meals-on-wheels. In recent years a stronger emphasis has been placed in many countries on care in the community, and more especially care in the older person's own home, commonly referred to as home care or domiciliary care, as opposed to institutional care (Scharf and Wenger, 1995).

This shift to care in the community and in the home has been slow to evolve but is now commonly and firmly promoted by policy makers and advocates of 'ageing in place', including older persons who, for the most part, have a preference for home care. In the light of population ageing, changes in family structures, an increase in women's labour market participation rates and the perceived unsuitability and high cost of institutional care, the challenge of providing adequate community care has become a policy concern of great importance. While the *proportion* of people in the older age groups in need of care appears to be declining, at least in some countries and some population groups (see, Fries, 2003, for instance), the *absolute number* of older people requiring care will increase. Most countries have made the decision at least in principle that, whenever possible, such care should take place in the older person's home. While it is certainly ill-advised to make overly pessimistic predictions about the availability of help and care from informal sources, there can be little doubt that the demand for *formal* home care services is set to increase significantly. In this context, it is important to understand the ways in which home care is organised, financed and delivered to older people in different policy contexts.

The explicit focus of this book, therefore, lies in the allocation, organisation and quality assurance systems of formal domiciliary (in-home) care services. This book compares the main features of domiciliary care policies for the older population in three contexts, namely, Denmark, the state of California in the United States and Germany. This introductory chapter is divided into four sections. First, it will outline the main frameworks and classifications that have been developed to assist in the comparative analysis of welfare states and social care. Second, it will provide a more detailed discussion on definitions of 'home care'. Third, it will highlight the complexities of undertaking cross-country analysis of social care and outline the approach taken in this book to analysing home care in the three different policy contexts. The final section outlines the structure of the book.

'USEFUL SIMPLIFICATIONS' OF WELFARE AND SOCIAL CARE SYSTEMS

The development and use of regime classifications, which are intended to serve as 'useful simplifications of reality', has by now a long history in the area of social policy research, particularly as it relates to transfer payments, that is, the benefits that the state pays to people who are affected by various 'social risks' such as unemployment, sickness and retirement. The first systematic attempt at general welfare state classification was undertaken by Titmuss (1974), who identified three distinct social policy models: the residual welfare model, the industrial achievement–performance model and the institutional redistributive model. This typology was considerably refined by Esping-Andersen (1990), who developed a welfare state classification based on levels of decommodification and social stratification provided across different welfare states, which took into account both the scale and structure of provision. He initially identified three distinct welfare state regimes as follows: the social-democratic model (Nordic countries); the continental or state corporatist model (for example, Germany, the Netherlands); and the liberal (Anglo-Saxon) model (for example, the UK). A fourth category – the Southern European model – to incorporate Italy, Spain, Portugal and Greece was subsequently added (Ferrera, 1996).

While welfare state regime classifications in relation to social protection and social transfer (cash benefit) payments are well established and widely applied, the same cannot be said of the area of social care provision. It has been argued that existing welfare state classifications are not entirely satisfactory in trying to understand variations across social care systems. This is because the field of social care is more complex and varied than that of cash benefits. In addition, regime classifications have tended to ignore some central features of social care, such as the extensive reliance in many countries on informal care (see, for instance, Anttonen and Sipilä, 1996; Esping-Andersen, 1999; Lewis, 2000). As Daly (2000, p. 37) points out '[e]ven in the most advanced welfare states, caring is never completely provided in the formal (professional) settings'. A good starting-point in constructing social care regimes is an acknowledgement that remarkably little is known about even the most basic aspects of informal care, such as the quantity of care and who provides it. Even the formal care services sector tends to be a complex field of research, as these services are often organised in a decentralised way. Additionally, in many countries data have to be collated from a range of different sources (whereas data on income transfers tend to be available from a single, centralised source). These problems are inevitably magnified when trying to compile data from a wide range of countries, although progress has recently been made in this regard (for instance, see OECD, 2005, for cross-national data on long-term care of older people).

Following the recognition that the three worlds of welfare capitalism are not entirely satisfactory for the purposes of classifying (and understanding) social care systems, a number of valuable attempts have been made to develop systematic ways of thinking about social care. Steps towards identifying services as a separate area of policy analysis were initially taken by Kohl (1981). Kohl's analysis of social expenditure and investment in services *vis-à-vis* cash benefits or transfers led him to highlight the dichotomy between 'service states' and 'transfer states'. The former tend to be coterminous with the Scandinavian countries, and the latter with continental corporatist welfare states (see also Kautto, 2002).

Alber (1995) recommends that the supply of social services to older people be analysed and compared using three variables: first, expenditure on such services; second, the number of residential and domiciliary care services; and third, the take-up rate of these services. However, the difficulty involved in obtaining accurate national representative statistics in relation to these areas tends to restrict analysis to countries that are more advanced in the collection of such statistics. Furthermore, while this information is useful, it does not elucidate the reasons for the variation between different social care systems. To explain this variation, Alber recommends further analysis of the respective systems under four broad headings: the regulatory structure, the financial structure, the structure of supply and the degree of consumer power.

In their work, Anttonen and Sipilä (1996, p. 87) set out to 'bring social care services into the domain of comparative social policy research' arguing that '[c]omparative research into social care services has not, as yet, made very impressive progress'. Drawing on small-scale empirical analysis of care services for children and older people, and on data on women's labour market participation rates, they identified two distinct models of social care services: the Scandinavian model of public services and the (Mediterranean) family care model. Two other, more tentative, models were also identified. These were the British means-tested model and the Central European subsidiarity model.

Drawing on these classifications and on data relating to developments in the 1990s in France, Spain, England, Sweden and Germany, Timonen (2005) identified three broad paradigms in the area of long-term care services for older people. The first of these is the statist paradigm, where the state takes extensive responsibility for financing and providing long-term care. The second is the familial/individualist paradigm, where families and individuals are responsible for financing long-term care and where services available through the state are means-tested and limited to a small proportion of the older population. In the third, referred to as 'state pays, others provide' paradigm, the state funds all or part of the costs of care while multiple players engage in the delivery of services (family, voluntary and private sector). In other words, there is a clear 'purchaser–provider' division. The parallels between these paradigms and two of the four models identified by Anttonen and Sipilä are clear; the family care and means-tested models are here collapsed into one (the familial/individualist model).

To date, the model developed by Anttonen and Sipilä arguably remains the single most useful and illuminating one, although it is clear, and explicitly stated by the authors themselves, that further work is needed. It is, of course, slightly ironic that efforts to develop a social care classification, which started with a critique of the three worlds of welfare capitalism, have to date produced classifications that are not entirely dissimilar from that developed by Esping-Andersen: the parallels between the Nordic welfare state regime and the Scandinavian social care model are evident, as are the similarities between the corporatist welfare state and the Central European subsidiarity models, and between the means-tested social care and the liberal welfare state models. Despite the fact that different variables are used, the resulting framework is astonishingly similar to Esping-Andersen's classification: surprisingly little has been made of this similarity in the literature. The analysis in this book shows that existing frameworks are helpful in elucidating the complexity of social care of older people in one particular context, that is, the domiciliary or home care setting. At the same time, however, it is of limited value in trying to capture the recent dynamics of change in this policy area.

Cross-country comparisons of social care regimes can yield valuable information, such as highlighting points of convergence between different systems and emerging trends. Positive and negative aspects and outcomes of particular systems can also be ascertained. As Kröger (2001, p. 11) asserts, 'comparative research on care for older people has considerable relevance for national policy making in sketching the alternatives, in showing their prospects and potential pitfalls'. This, of course, is not tantamount to arguing that care policies can or should be transplanted either in full or in part.

DEFINING DOMICILIARY CARE/HOME CARE

The generic term 'home care' is often used interchangeably with the term 'domiciliary care'. Cullen et al. (2004) offer a useful typology that helps to define the parameters of domiciliary or home care for the purposes of this book. According to their typology, care can be broken down into four categories:

- Practical: for example, domestic tasks such as preparing a meal, cleaning the house and doing shopping.
- Personal: for example, washing and bathing, help with getting dressed and providing continence care.
- Monitoring/supervision: for example, of persons with dementia who may be confused when using appliances or in danger of wandering.
- Care management: providing support through management activities such as liaising with health professionals and coordinating care services.

Persons who require domiciliary care services usually have a limitation in 'activities of daily living' (ADL) such as washing, dressing or eating, and/or in 'instrumental activities of daily living' (IADL) such as shopping, cleaning or meal preparation. Home carers typically work in a dual capacity. They deliver light domestic care (assistance with IADL) including food preparation, light housework and companionship services such as accompanying clients to medical appointments. They also provide personal care (assistance with ADL) such as helping the older person in and out of bed, assistance with dressing, prompting medication, bathing, application of ointments, showering and grooming. Whether or not an older person with ADL/IADL difficulties is eligible for state-funded domiciliary care services varies according to the regulations in a specific country: in some instances, eligibility is determined on the basis of income and assets, in others, it is the degree of ADL limitations that determines eligibility; there are also systems where a combination of both means and functional ability is used to determine eligibility.

'Home care' or 'domiciliary care' has different meanings in different systems. While a distinction can be made between medical and non-medical or social care services the focus of this study is on non-medical domiciliary care. Nevertheless, it is important to note that in practice such categories are often blurred, as illustrated by the area of paramedics. In the United States for instance, home carers in California's largest home care programme, the In-Home Supportive Services (IHSS), can perform paramedical tasks such as dispensing medication, dressing wounds and administering injections; in Germany, informal carers who are paid via the long-term care insurance

(LTCI) programme can deliver paramedical services; while in Denmark, paramedical care services are the preserve of qualified nurses.

Terminology surrounding home care varies across and within different countries. For example, Tester (1996, p.5) points out that the concept of 'community care' as used in the UK, is commonly referred to as 'community-based long-term care' in the US. Also, in the US home carers can be called 'home-makers', 'caregivers' or 'providers'. In Ireland they are frequently called 'home-helps' or personal care assistants or attendants (Timonen et al., 2006). In the UK and Australia they are called 'carers', while in India and some other countries they are called 'care-takers' (WHO, 2002). Similarly, whereas home care recipients are typically referred to as 'consumers' in the United States, in other countries they are referred to as 'home care beneficiaries'. In this review, for the purposes of clarity and uniformity, the workers are generally referred to as 'carers' or 'home carers' and the receiver of the domiciliary services as the 'home care recipient' or 'beneficiary'.

The term 'informal care' is used in this book to denote care provided by family members, neighbours or friends. While the focus of this book lies in formal domiciliary care, that is, care provided by paid workers, it is naturally not possible to consider the realm of domiciliary care without acknowledging the fact that even where formal carers are involved, they usually work alongside informal, generally family, carers. As Abrahamson et al. (2005, p. 12) note, 'the provision of welfare in any modern society is, in fact, always a combination of market, public and civil societal interventions into private individuals' lives'. The provision of informal care is thus of paramount importance in any discussion on domiciliary care since the support networks of the majority of older people are dominated by kin. Furthermore, as Wellin (2006, p. 210) points out, 'one's ability to remain at home and avoid institutionalisation is shaped by support networks as much as by health status per se'.

The availability of public social care services greatly influences the demand for and nature of informal care. Countries with more developed formal social care systems and countries that do not specify legal family obligations to care for ageing family members in need of care tend to be less reliant on informal care (for a discussion of this 'substitution effect', see Chapter 8). Increasingly, countries are beginning to formally recognise (and encourage) the contribution of informal caregivers, either by paying them a cash benefit, in some cases equivalent to the wages of a contracted home care worker, or by providing money to the care recipient to pay the informal caregiver of their choice. In addition, social security entitlements, such as pensions and holiday pay are in some instances given to these informal carers. However, in a number of countries these rights and entitlements are not extended to close relatives such as a spouse, a daughter or a son, and can be channelled only to non-family members such as neighbours, friends or other informal contacts.

FOCUS OF THIS BOOK

Regardless of which of the welfare state regime classifications discussed above is applied, the three cases selected broadly adhere to three different 'regimes'. The United States adheres to the liberal welfare regime, Germany to the corporatist and Denmark to the social-democratic regime. In terms of social care regimes or paradigms, the three systems also align with three distinct 'clusters'. The selection of these three cases reflects the decision to opt for 'different' systems, with a view to teasing out the main differences between them in the 'subfield' of domiciliary social care for older people.

As discussed in more detail in Chapter 8, thinking about care policies in the light of these classifications is helpful up to a point. However, it became clear in the course of the research that the traditional social care regime classifications have in many instances been unsettled by recent developments within each of the care regimes, and in some cases their use distracted attention away from the areas of similarity or convergence.

Every attempt has been made to keep the discussion on each of the three countries broad and, hopefully, of general or comparative interest. It should be noted, however, that in the case of the United States it was necessary to focus on one single state because interstate differences in social care are very extensive. The State of California was chosen as the focus because it has one of the largest state-plan programmes in the US; while not providing a perfect 'microcosm' of the complexity of social care in the US, the analysis of this programme none the less alerts the reader to many of the key and distinctive features of care policy in the that country. This book, therefore, presents a comparative analysis of the key aspects of: (i) formal domiciliary care financed through LTCI in Germany, (ii) IHSS in California and (iii) the public domiciliary care service in Denmark.

The domiciliary care sector is constantly changing with new amendments and legislative reforms introduced, often at a rapid pace. To acquire up-to-date information on the three systems, 25 key persons including administrators, interest group representatives and academics/experts were interviewed in Denmark, Germany and the State of California between October 2005 and March 2006. The purpose of these interviews was twofold: first, to acquire a comprehensive understanding of the delivery structure of these systems, and second, to qualitatively explore the perceptions interviewees had of the strengths and weaknesses of their respective domiciliary care systems. Extracts from a number of these interviews have been incorporated into the three main country chapters to reflect the opinions of a select group of individuals within each of the three care regimes.

Most comparative analyses of social care systems approach the topic at a macro level, thus neglecting the way in which the system functions at the coalface of social care provision. While analysis of the institutional frameworks, financial and delivery structures and the issue of consumer power provide useful insights into the three care systems, a specific focus on the delivery of services on the ground and the day-to-day reality of domiciliary care service was also deemed necessary in order to gain a better insight into the respective care regimes. While not in a position to do a comprehensive analysis of domiciliary care services as perceived by both workers and care recipients, an attempt was made to gain a cursory insight into the dynamics of the care relationship in each of the three systems. To this end, three observation days were arranged with a domiciliary care worker in each of the three countries. Naturally, short observation exercises are far from ideal in teasing out the many complexities and issues that arise in the context of home care (see Sarantakos, 2005, for a discussion on the advantages and disadvantages of observational methods). However, it offers a first step in challenging the assumption that comparative analysis of domiciliary care systems can take place only at the macro or institutional/policy level.

In addition to these primary sources, secondary sources were extensively consulted, prior to and after the interviews and observation exercises. Secondary sources included government reports, books, journal articles and websites and were used to substantiate and validate the information gleaned from the primary sources. Drawing on both primary and secondary sources, the book highlights some of the main policy, organisational and operational differences between the three domiciliary care systems. The methodological approach adopted may not have made it possible to surmount all of the difficulties that arise when conducting comparative research. However, it is believed that the use of both primary and secondary sources serves to strengthen the analysis. We hope that it makes for an insightful and interesting review of policy development in an increasingly important subfield of domiciliary social care for older people.

CHAPTER STRUCTURE

This book is organised into eight chapters. Chapter 2 provides background data that serves to illustrate the different contexts in which the three domiciliary care systems operate. With a view to outlining the parameters within which each system operates, it provides an overview of key variables such as age profile, life expectancy at birth, old-age dependency ratios, number of persons living alone and spending on health and long-term care. Chapters 3, 4 and 5 analyse the domiciliary care policies and practices in

Denmark, the United States (California) and Germany, respectively. Each of these three chapters follows a similar structure in reviewing the key institutional features of the domiciliary care systems. Drawing on Alber (1995), the review of the three systems is largely based on (i) the regulatory structure, (ii) the financing structure, (iii) the delivery structure and (iv) the degree of consumer power, choice and direction within the respective long-term care programmes.

Chapter 6 describes the observation exercises that took place in the three contexts. It extends the discussion on domiciliary care from the policy and administrative elements of the systems to the home and the care worker and care recipient and compares the observation exercises conducted in each country. Chapter 7 provides a comparative analysis of domiciliary care. It attempts to draw together the preceding four chapters by taking a comparative approach to key themes and policy areas such as eligibility assessments, quality, workforce issues, consumer direction and informal care (as supported from public funds). Chapter 8 concludes by outlining the lessons for future research in the area and the most pressing research and policy challenges to be addressed in the field of domiciliary care for older people.

2. Setting the Scene: The Context for Domiciliary Care in the Three Countries

This chapter explores a number of key indicators which may affect to varying degrees demands for long-term care services in Denmark, the United States and Germany. The indicators chosen are life expectancy at birth; the age profile in each country, that is, the proportion of the population aged 65 years and over, and 80 years and over; dependency ratios and living arrangements of older persons in each of the three countries. The chapter then goes on to examine public and private expenditure on health and long-term care and the use of formal long-term care services. These variables were chosen as they were deemed to have a significant influence on both the current contexts of the three domiciliary care systems and, in some instances, the future demand for care that these regimes may have to confront. The data contained in this chapter are, for the most part, obtained from the Organisation for Economic Co-operation and Development (OECD) and the Population Division of the United Nations.

LIFE EXPECTANCY AT BIRTH

Increasing life expectancy is one of the driving forces behind ageing populations. Life expectancy at birth has increased at a remarkably consistent rate in the majority of developed countries due to a combination of improved medical treatment and improved socio-economic and environmental conditions. The average life expectancy at birth across Germany, Denmark and the United States is fairly similar, although the population of Germany fares slightly better. Overall, life expectancy at birth is one year and two months longer for German citizens as compared to either US or Danish citizens (OECD, 2005). German women can expect on average to live one year and six months longer than their US counterparts and one year and ten months longer than their Danish counterparts (ibid.). For men, life expectancy at birth is also highest for German males who, on average, will live one year and one month longer than their US counterparts and nine months longer than their Danish counterparts (ibid.) (see Figure 2.1).

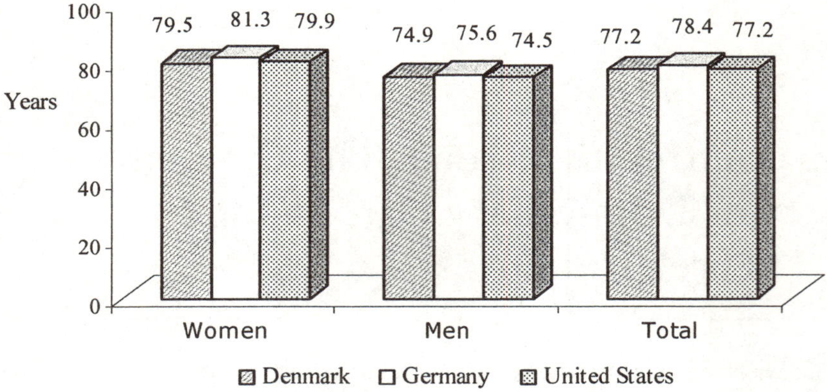

Source: OECD (2005 Chart HE 1), www.oecd.org/els/social/indicators/SAG.

Figure 2.1 Life expectancy at birth in Denmark, Germany and the United States, 2002

AGE PROFILE

At present, Germany is the oldest of the three countries with 16.4 per cent of its population aged 65 years and over. Denmark is next with 14.8 per cent of its population aged 65 and over, while the United States is considerably younger with only 12.4 per cent of its population aged over 65 (see Figure 2.2).

Currently, the three countries have fairly similar percentages of persons aged 80 years and over. The oldest old-age group is proportionately largest in Denmark, with 4 per cent of its population aged 80 or over, followed by Germany with 3.7 per cent and the United States with 3.3 per cent (see Figure 2.2). The predicted growth of this cohort is particularly relevant for any discussion on long-term care, since it is this population that is more likely to require greater levels of often high-intensity care. It is estimated that the number of persons in this oldest old-age category will rise in each of the three countries in the coming decades, but to varying degrees. In the United States it is estimated that the number of persons aged 80 years and over will rise by almost 20 million by 2050, while in Germany it will rise by 5 million (United Nations Population Division, 2000). However, the growth rate, of the over-80s population in Denmark is not predicted to be as pronounced, with estimates that it will grow by less than 10 per cent by approximately 2020 (European Commission, 2003).

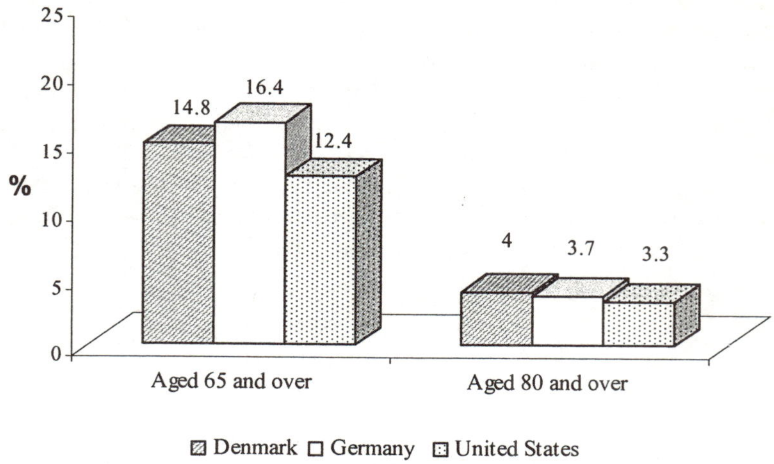

Source: OECD (2005, Table A.1, p. 101).

Figure 2.2 People aged 65 years and over and aged 80 and over as a percentage of the population, 2000

OLD-AGE DEPENDENCY RATIOS

The 'old-age dependency ratio' is a simple and widely used demographic indicator in comparative analysis. The frequent use of these ratios is perhaps largely due to the fact that they are easy to understand, easy to compute and easy to obtain. The old-age dependency ratio refers to the number of older people (aged 65 years and over) divided by the working-age population (aged 15 to 64 years). In 2000, the ratio was highest for Germany at 24 per cent, followed by Denmark at 22 per cent and the United States at 19 per cent. Projections made by the OECD (2006) predict that old-age dependency ratios will increase substantially in the future. The ratio is predicted to double to 49 per cent in Germany, to rise to 42 per cent in Denmark, and to reach 32 per cent in the United States (see Figure 2.3).

Old-age dependency ratios are only useful up to a point. Although sometimes used to give an indication of reliance on social protection and need for long-term care, they give only a crude indication of the balance between the older 'dependent' and the younger 'active' or 'productive' segments of the population on the basis of chronological age. The ratios fail to take account of the fact that the majority of older people do not and will not require continuous or extensive assistance with activities of daily living and, indeed, may not require formal long-term care services. In addition, their value may become increasingly less important, if a greater number of people are given the opportunity to work beyond the age of 65 years in the coming decades. Furthermore, their use can at times lead to an exaggerated sense of crisis (Pierce, 2006) and create the catastrophic impression of a demographic time-bomb (Pacolet, 2001). 'Dependency' is a construct that can be measured in varying ways. For example, Pacolet defines dependency in terms of four dimensions: physical, mental, social and economic. When viewed in this way, it seems that dependency tends to appear later in life than is the case when chronological age is used, as in old-age dependency ratios (ibid.).

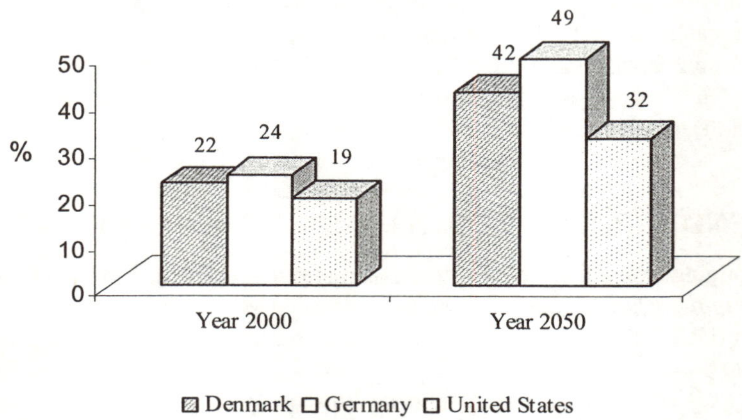

Note: Population aged 65 and over as a percentage of population aged 15–69.
Source: OECD (2006, Chart GE 2.1), www.oecd.org/els/social/indicators/SAG.

Figure 2.3 Actual and predicted old-age dependency ratios

LIVING ARRANGEMENTS AND SINGLE-OCCUPANCY HOUSEHOLDS

The living arrangements of older people may affect, among other things, health status, the availability of informal care, health behaviours and access to material resources (see Berkman and Glass, 2000). Generally, persons living alone will be at a greater risk of vulnerability. Making direct cross-country comparisons regarding the number of persons aged 65 and over living alone is, however, difficult due to the fact that frequently classifications are based on different age ranges. Statistics available from the European Commission (2003) indicate that, in 1995, 36 per cent of the Danish population aged between 65 and 79 years lived in single-occupancy households, compared with 30 per cent of the German population. These figures are considerably higher for persons aged 80 years and over: 62 per cent in Denmark and 52 per cent in Germany. Figures available from the US Census (2005) use a different age classification, that is, 65 to 74 years. According to these figures, 37 per cent of 65–74 year olds in the US live in single-occupancy households, while 55 per cent of persons aged 75 years and over live alone. These figures would suggest that proportionally more people in Denmark live in single-occupancy households and that the availability of 'in-house' informal care is lower in Denmark where a larger proportion of the older population lives alone. It is not clear what the exact relationship is between a person's living arrangements and the need for formal long-term care services (Grundy, 2001). However, research has indicated that those who live alone are more likely to receive formal care services than those who live in co-residence households (ibid.). On the basis of this, the current demand for formal care would be higher in Denmark than in either Germany or the United States.

EXPENDITURE ON HEALTH AND LONG-TERM CARE

In examining expenditure on health and long-term care in a comparative context, it is more illuminating to examine spending relative to gross domestic product (GDP) than to focus on nominal expenditure levels. It is also useful to distinguish between public and private health expenditure. Public expenditure includes all costs incurred by public institutions, regional government, municipalities, sickness funds or old-age funds. Private spending refers to private out-of-pocket payments or payments by private long-term care insurance funds. Figures from the OECD (2006) indicate that both public and private sources play a crucial role in financing the US health care system, with 44.9 per cent of all health expenditure coming from public sources and 55.1 per cent coming from private sources. Denmark has the lowest proportion of private expenditure on health at 17.1 per cent in comparison with 82.9 per cent of expenditure coming from public sources (ibid.). Similarly, in Germany, the bulk of expenditure is from public sources at 78.5 per cent compared with 21.5 from private sources (see Figure 2.4).

An examination of public expenditure on health in the three countries shows that spending in both Germany and the United States has increased since 1980, from 6.8 to 8.6 per cent of GDP in Germany and 3.6 to 6.6 per cent of GDP in the United States (OECD, 2006). It is interesting to note, however, that health expenditure in Denmark has been decreasing since 1980; in 1980, 8 per cent of its GDP was spent on health, while in 2002 this had decreased to 7.3 per cent (ibid.) (see Figure 2.5).

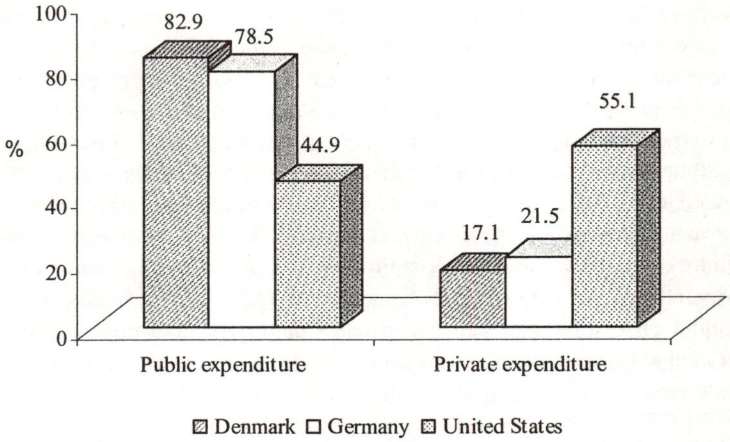

Source: OECD (2006, Table Health spending and resources), www.oecd.org/document/62/0,2340,en_2649_34489_2345918_1_1_1_1,00. html.

Figure 2.4 Public and private expenditure on health as a percentage of total expenditure on health

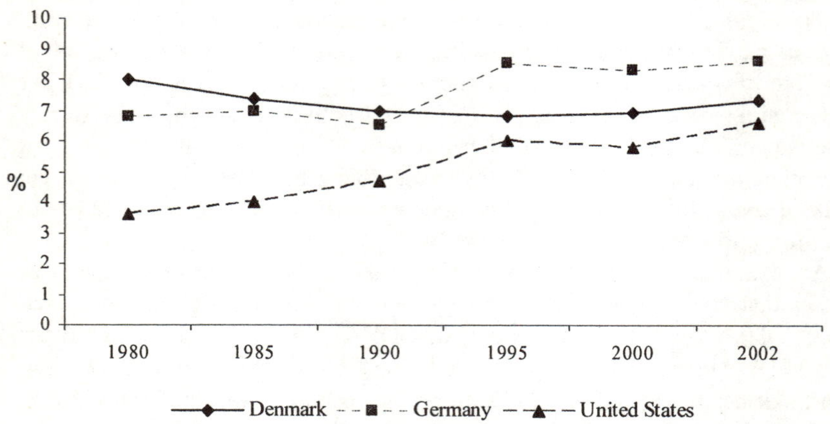

Source: OECD (2006, Table HE4.2), www.oecd.org/els/social/indicators/SAG.

Figure 2.5 Public expenditure on health as a percentage of GDP, 1980–2002

However, not all expenditure, on health goes to older people. In Denmark, long-term care services are financed through the social services budget, while in Germany they are financed from care insurance funds. For this reason, it is necessary to focus explicitly on spending on long-term care. Figures on long-term care expenditure in the three countries reveal some noteworthy differences. According to the OECD (2006), Denmark spends approximately 1.8 per cent of its GDP on long-term care, compared with 1.35 per cent in Germany and 1.29 per cent in the United States. In the case of Denmark it was not possible to differentiate between spending on institutional care and home care. In Germany, public expenditure on home care was marginally lower than institutional care expenditure, 0.43 and 0.52 per cent of GDP, respectively. In the United States, too, public spending on institutional care was higher than expenditure on home care, 0.58 per cent compared with 0.17 per cent of GDP.

Private expenditure on home care was highest in the United States at 0.16 per cent of GDP, compared with only 0.04 per cent of GDP in Germany and 0.1 per cent in Denmark. Private expenditure on institutional care, however, was fairly similar in Germany and the United States; figures on private institutional care expenditure were not available for Denmark but can be assumed to be very low (see Table 2.1).

Table 2.1 Public and private expenditure on long-term care as percentage of GDP

	Germany (2000)	United States (2000)	Denmark (2003)
		Total Expenditure	
Home care	0.47	0.33	1.8e
Institutional	0.88	0.96	
Total	1.35	1.29	1.8e
		Public expenditure	
Home care	0.43	0.17	1.7e
Institutional	0.52	0.58	
Total	0.95	0.74	1.7e
		Private expenditure	
Home care	0.04	0.16	0.10 e
Institutional	0.36	0.39	NA
Total	0.40	0.54	NA

Note: e = estimate.

Sources: Germany and United States: OECD (2005, Table 1.2, p. 26). Denmark: OECD (2006, Total expenditure on long-term nursing care at home % gross domestic product).

USE OF FORMAL LONG-TERM CARE SERVICES

The availability of long-term care services, whether they are institutional or community services, private or public, may reflect the emphasis that a particular country places on formal long-term care services and, to a lesser degree, demand for such services. Figure 2.6 below illustrates that the proportion of the older population receiving formal home care services (both public and private services) is largest in Denmark at 20.3 per cent. This contrasts with 16 per cent in the United States and 9.6 per cent in Germany.

When figures relating to institutional care are compared, Denmark again has the highest proportion of its older population (7 per cent) in receipt of institutional care. This figure includes modern and innovative forms of residential care such as independent living in sheltered housing and senior citizens' homes, and hence does not give a precise estimate of 'traditional' nursing home use. As Chapter 3 will show, the percentage of persons who are receiving care in traditional institutional settings in Denmark is likely to be low given the fact that priority is placed on the delivery of services in sheltered housing dwellings. It is estimated that 5.7 per cent of the over-65 population in the United States and 6.8 per cent of the German over-65 population are in institutional care. Once again, these figures are not broken down according to the specific type of residential care; such information would obviously be highly relevant as the 'traditional' nursing home setting can be very different from, for instance, assisted living complexes. These figures, however, highlight the fact that availability of formal long-term care services is highest in Denmark and perhaps reflect the emphasis placed on the public provision of long-term care services and that such are universally available for free to all Danish citizens.

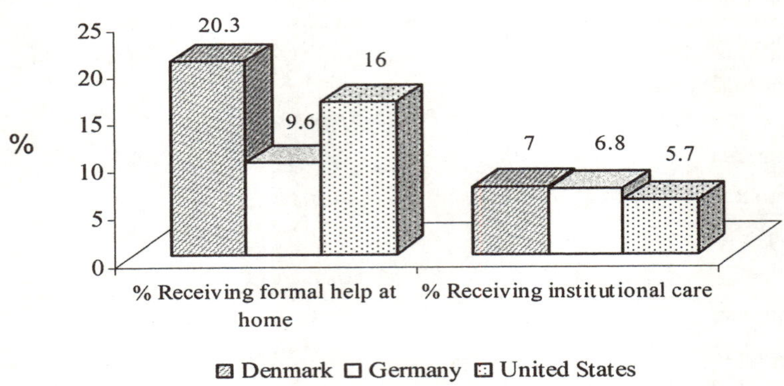

Source: Jacobzone (2000, Table 2, www.isuma.net/v01n02/jacobzone/jacobzone_e.shtml)

Figure 2.6 Percentage of population aged 65 years and over receiving formal care, by care setting

CONCLUSIONS

Many factors can in varying ways influence the demand for publicly funded domiciliary care. Establishing the main influencing factors and acquiring comparable statistical information about these key indicators, however, is a difficult challenge. The variables outlined above are only some of the factors that may impact upon the demand for long-term care services. Factors such as income and material resources of older people, family and social supports, provision and receipt of informal support by kin and social contacts (Grundy, 2001) and the organisation and provision of formal long-term care services (Pacolet, 2001) are also highly relevant and will continue to reflect and shape the three long-term care regimes under examination. Furthermore, issues such as improved health and environmental conditions, development of assisting technologies and increasing numbers of older people in the workforce will impact on the pressure placed on long-term care systems.

The data provided above suggest that the three countries face many similar social challenges, such as an ageing age profile, a growth in the over-80s population, increasing life expectancies and increases in old-age dependency ratios. Such major social changes are likely to impact on the demand for domiciliary care services. If this is the case, the important question of 'who' gets care and 'how much' care a person gets is likely to become of increasing relevance. Currently, public and private spending on health differs significantly across the three countries, with people in the United States having to cover more of the costs of their health and social care privately than citizens in either Germany or Denmark. Interestingly, while aggregate spending on long-term care is fairly similar, as the following chapters will show, the coverage and level of publicly provided or financed provision is drastically different. With this in mind the following three chapters attempt to elucidate the current institutional structures and realities of the home care systems in Denmark, the United States and Germany.

3. Formal Domiciliary Care in Denmark

This chapter discusses the regulatory, financial and delivery structure of the Danish domiciliary care system and describes the key legislative changes that have occurred in recent years. These changes have had enormous implications for both the municipalities' role as providers of domiciliary care and the ability of home care recipients to exercise consumer choice with respect to the care they receive. The chapter argues that these changes mark a new departure in the Danish welfare state, where transparency and an emphasis on cost monitoring and quality control have become increasingly important.

Denmark is often referred to as a 'model country' in the area of care services for older people. Of all of the European countries, Denmark has the highest provision of home care for those aged 65 and over, providing on average nearly twice as many hours of home help as its closest competitor, Sweden (Stuart and Weinrich, 2001).[1] It was one of the first countries to adopt a community care policy and since the 1970s has favoured care in the home over institutional care. Together with this, Denmark has a long tradition of public welfare provision, which can be dated to the eighteenth century. According to Vallgårda et al. (2001, p. 10):

> [T]he roots of the Danish welfare state date back to the eighteenth century, long before the emergence of social democratic parties and organized philanthropy, and the fact that many Scandinavian public authorities were also benefactors may explain why attitudes to the state are often more positive in Scandinavia than in other western European countries.

Present-day Danish policy relating to older people is based on three principles, namely, (i) continuity in the individual's life; (ii) the use of personal resources and (iii) autonomy and influence on one's own circumstances (Ministry of Social Affairs, 2002). By law, home care is to be provided to those who have regular difficulty with daily living activities. Family circumstances (typically the absence or presence of a healthy spouse) are taken into consideration only in relation to domestic help. In addition to being needs and rights-based, home care services are universal, which means that they are free at the point of use.[2] Apart from a short period when fees were payable, domiciliary care has been free to all persons requiring assistance on an ongoing basis since 1 July 1989 (Holstein et al., 1991).

REGULATORY STRUCTURE

When legislation on home care in Denmark was first introduced in 1949 it was means-tested and targeted towards families with children (Holstein et al., 1991). However, legislation introduced in 1958 specified that the municipality must provide assistance to older people with a view to helping them to continue living at home. The passing of the Social Services Act in 1972 further extended the responsibility of municipalities for decisions concerning care of older people and obliged municipalities to both determine need and provide home care services to all those in need of domiciliary care. Under the Act, the basis of an older person's eligibility for help is determined by his/her level of disability or care needs. A fundamental principle underpinning the Act is that help has to be seen in terms of promoting self-reliance and independence, as well as facilitating daily activities and enhancing the quality of life of older people. Thus since the 1970s, regulation and administration of health care provision has been largely decentralised, with the majority of the responsibility for the financing and provision of health care (including domiciliary care) entrusted to the county and municipal authorities.

The Social Services Act, 1972, still provides the legislative basis for public social services, which includes domiciliary care. The Act promotes a unified, decentralised social care system. It requires municipalities[3] to provide the necessary number of social services to its citizens. Each municipality makes its own policy with regard to provision, and decides the number of places deemed to be necessary or sufficient. While the law states that the municipality must do whatever is possible to keep a person in his/her own home, there are no formal minimum standards and the legislative specification of providing domiciliary care 'according to an individual's needs' is open to interpretation by the municipalities. The Social Services Act, 1972, has been amended a number of times so that the provision of home care, which was initially granted on a discretionary basis, has become an entitlement.

The Housing for the Elderly Act introduced in 1987 prohibited the building of new nursing homes. It also stipulated that specialist assisted living housing (*ældrebolig*) should be available to older people. Responsibility for the construction and control of access to these dwellings was conferred on the municipality (Lewinter, 2004). Additional legislation enacted in 1997 specified that each assisted living dwelling is to have its own food-making facilities and accessible bathroom and can measure up to 62 square metres for a single person (ibid.). The effects of the 1987 legislation have been considerable. Traditional nursing homes have closed at an approximate rate of 10 per cent per year (Meijer et al., 2000), while the number of assisted living dwellings increased from 3,356 in 1987 to 37,899 in 2001 (Lewinter, 2004).

At a national level, the federal government or Ministry of Social Affairs is limited in its capacity to influence the delivery of social care services and is only permitted to supervise and advise the counties and municipalities in this regard (Vallgårda et al., 2001). In recent years, however, the federal government has introduced a number of changes in order to bring about a somewhat more formalised, uniform, transparent and streamlined domiciliary care system throughout the country. On 1 January 2003, a new law entitled 'Greater Choice for the Provider' was introduced. The purpose of this legislation was multifaceted: while still entrusting local authorities with responsibility for financing, supervision and ensuring that there was an adequate supply of domiciliary care, the provision and supervision of these services were separated for the first time. While municipalities retained responsibility for organising the provision of social services, services for the first time were to be delivered by both the public and private sectors.[4] Up to 2001, local municipalities were the only providers of publicly financed domiciliary care. The principal implication of the 2003 legislation was that private domiciliary care providers could now compete with the municipality to offer publicly financed domiciliary care. A report from the Ministry of Social Affairs (2002, p. 46) explains it in the following terms:

> [T]he free choice of service provider obliges local authorities to ensure, in so far as possible, that older people have a selection of several service providers from which to choose. The local authority may either enter into agreements with all service providers wishing to offer personal and practical help and assistance in compliance with the price and quality requirement stipulated by the local authority or it may invite tenders and subsequently award contracts to a pre-defined number of service providers (2–5 providers).

This law thus conferred on the municipality greater administrative and regulatory powers and served to differentiate between the municipalities' functions as purchasers and regulators of services, on the one hand, and as providers of services, on the other (see Figure 3.1). These changes were intended to improve efficiency and enable the municipality to focus less attention on direct service provision and instead to take overall responsibility for regulation and supervision of service delivery. Another rationale for this reallocation of responsibility and the introduction of new social care markets was that it permitted greater financial objectivity and accountability. This new realignment and new mode of service delivery and regulation is not only linked to the issue of quality of care, but is also closely related to efforts at a national level to reduce or contain costs relating to care (Csonksa and Boll, 2000).

The redefinition of the role of the municipalities and the move towards subcontracting care out to private providers is generally regarded as part of a new political ideology geared towards the restructuring of the Danish welfare state in general (see Green-Pedersen, 2002). New management initiatives (New Public Management) have been introduced to bring about greater levels of transparency and cost-control mechanisms. A public servant interviewed in the Ministry of Social Affairs explained that the reasoning behind this new legislation has been the desire to improve service quality:

It's also about increasing competition to improve quality. We have seen from recent studies that the public providers are getting more focused on delivering the same care worker [something which they had previously been criticised as failing to do]. It also makes the process more transparent . . . now you can see how the taxpayers' money is being spent on domiciliary care, what is the quality and how much care is available in each municipality. (Interviewee in the Ministry of Social Affairs)

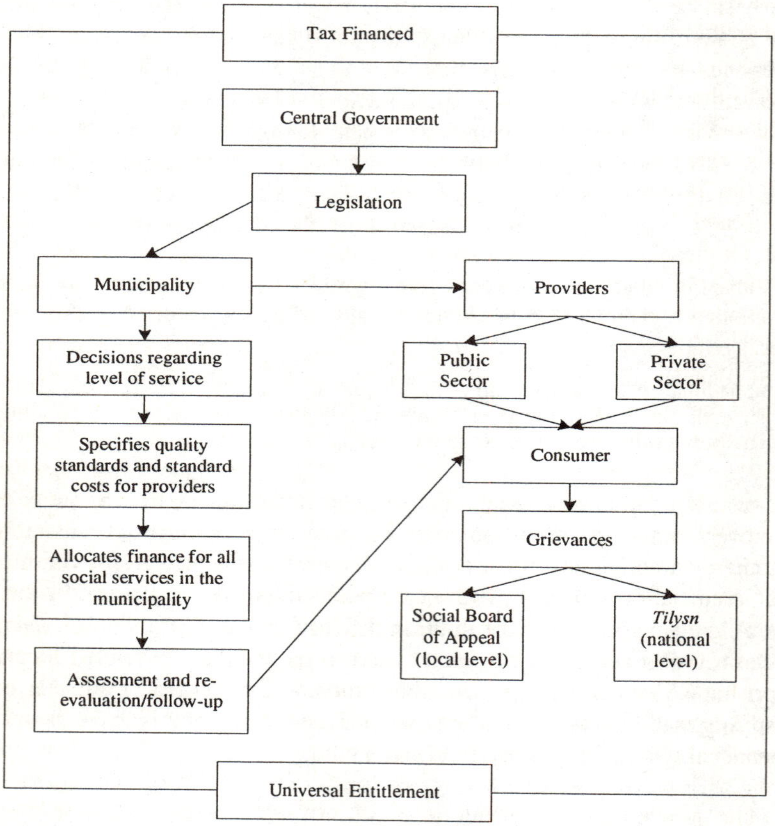

Figure 3.1 Home care in Denmark

According to a number of interviewees there appears to be a view that poor leadership among some of the public domiciliary care service providers prompted many of the municipalities to favour the new model of delivery. Furthermore, the public service model was deemed to be excessively top heavy and bureaucratic, so that, in many instances, home care workers did not get the support they required.

Despite the changes, responsibility for the provision of home care remains largely decentralised. Politicians within each of the municipalities specify the overall standard or 'service levels' within their jurisdiction. They both specify the criteria that domiciliary care providers must fulfil to be a supplier and determine the standard price for this service. In other words, the 'contracting out' of service provision takes place within a very clearly delineated and tightly controlled framework. Within this framework, the public sector, arguably, retains the predominant role in decision making and standard setting and even with regard to the determination of prices. Service-level agreements should be reviewed and updated annually by locally elected political representatives. However, the extent to which these annual reviews are conducted in all of the municipalities is questionable. For example, a study by Schultz-Larsen et al. (2004) found that 34 of the 36 municipalities researched had developed a quality list. Of these only 19 had revised the standards within a year, 13 had not revised the list in more than a year, two had not revised it for more than two years, while another two did not know when the standards had last been reviewed.

Local politicians who are responsible for the overall social services budget have to consider domiciliary care in the context of the sum total of social services that they are obliged to provide. This means that variations exist between municipalities in the provision of domiciliary care infrastructure. As Holstein et al. (1991, p. 43) point out, 'every local government "commune" must organize home help, but the amount is left open. As a consequence of the autonomy of local governments, the provision of home help services varies considerably from one to another'. Nevertheless, electoral mechanisms put pressure on municipal politicians to provide high-quality domiciliary care services (Alber, 1995). A growing proportion of the Danish electorate is aged over 65, which serves as a visible political lobby group that can put pressure on elected administrators to provide a satisfactory care infrastructure. This sentiment was relayed by a spokesperson interviewed in the Danish Trade Union of Public Employees (Forbendet af Offentligt Ansatte: FOA) who stated:

> [T]he people who are running for office, every fourth year, will have to be judged by the voters and even though domiciliary care is now outsourced they are responsible. So if they do not perform, they have to leave office and I would say that's a good thing about the system. (Interviewee in FOA)

A powerful financial incentive has been created aimed at ensuring a timely transition from hospital settings to community and other non-medical long-term care settings. Municipalities are penalised if they do not have suitable community care in place for a patient discharged from hospital. Where community care is not made available, the municipalities have to take responsibility for any additional hospital charges that may be incurred by the patient

(Vallgårda et al., 2001). This requirement is also extended to persons in need of specific domiciliary care services, that is, if the municipality does not have a specific service available (for example, night-time care), it is obliged to purchase this service from another region (Danish Ministry of the Interior and Health, 2004). Furthermore, all persons aged 70 years and over must receive a visit from the public health nurse within three days of hospital discharge.

The responsibility of the municipality is therefore extensive. By law, each municipality must ensure that adequate domiciliary care services are available within its jurisdiction. If required, the municipality must ensure that domiciliary care is available during the night, at weekends and during holidays. The service often combines home nursing care provided by a nurse and domiciliary care delivered by a domiciliary carer. With respect to the latter, the main priority is personal care, but it can also include help with housekeeping. Some municipalities provide help with cooking, laundry and shopping. In most municipalities house cleaning is available and is provided once or twice a fortnight depending on the needs of the care recipient. Services such as emergency help, which are available round-the-clock, as well as patient education and help in completing medical applications are also available from a public health nurse (Jarden and Jarden, 2002).

Eligibility Assessment

Access to domiciliary care is universal. In line with the statist paradigm of long-term care (see Timonen, 2005), the state does not expect the family to take the main responsibility for caregiving duties to an older family member. While consideration is given to the capacity and resources of a spouse in respect of the domiciliary care assessment, in principle, no consideration is given to the resources of additional family members or adult children not living in the house. Home care services are typically allocated in a preventive rather than a reactive (crisis) context, reflecting the overall aim of home care policies of averting or delaying the development of problems. Unlike the United States or Germany, the home care eligibility evaluation in Denmark is not measured by a universal assessment tool. Instead, each assessment considers the functional capacity of the individual in the light of the holistic needs and circumstances of the individual person. To this end, all home care recipients are awarded a care package designed to accommodate their unique care requirements.

Until the late 1990s the domiciliary care assessment was conducted by the domiciliary care manager or public service provider. However, as a result of criticisms voiced during the 1990s that this assessment was too subjective, dependent on the personality of the individual evaluator and the knowledge they had of the potential recipient, this arrangement was changed. To ensure more objectivity, the task of assessment was taken from the service provider and the new post of home care assessor was created. The assessor is now employed by the municipality as opposed to the service provider, is usually a qualified nurse and works full-time as a home care assessor. According to a researcher who has done extensive research on domiciliary care provision in Denmark and who was interviewed for the purpose of this review, the creation of the new role of assessor has caused some disquiet among public sector domiciliary care workers, who at times feel estranged from the assessor:

> [B]efore this purchasing–provider split, many domiciliary carers [in the public sector] felt the assessor was much closer to them. She was a nurse and often doing home nursing, so she knew a lot of clients and they often had the same offices next to each other so it was much more informal to go in and say 'Ms Jensen needs more care' and so on. Whereas now, you have to go through the leader of the team and make a request for more time and then document why you think the person needs more time and why their needs have changed and a lot are saying it's much more formal. Also, because you are dealing with a cohort of the population that doesn't have high education, they often have problems writing on the computer for instance, or just expressing themselves, or arguing a point. So for them to confront someone with a different education and status can be quite difficult. (Interview with Danish academic/researcher)

According to Danish law, the municipalities must process domiciliary care applications as quickly as possible and specify a minimum waiting period. In the study by Schultz-Larsen et al. (2004) municipalities were asked about the number of working days they allowed, first, between an application and a visit, and second, between a visit and delivery of services. Results indicated that requests were processed quickly. More specifically, requests for personal care were dealt with within three days by 19 of the 36 municipalities. Over and above this, 34 of the 36 municipalities had formal maximum periods within which the need for practical and personal help should be re-evaluated: 21 municipalities did this annually and 11 biannually.

In some areas there has been a reduction in the amount of care awarded by the municipalities. This reduction concerns domestic rather than personal care. A contentious issue surrounding discussions on the granting of home care relates to differences in how the care is awarded across municipalities and whether 'time' or a 'care task' is awarded. According to interviewees, in the past (five to ten years ago) care tended to be awarded in blocks of one hour, during which time the carer could complete a variety of tasks. More recently, however, there has been a visible reduction in the amount of time awarded, with time now typically awarded in blocks of 15, 25 or 45 minutes. In most areas, care is awarded in such units of time, with a specified number of minutes allocated to a task. Such regimented allocation of time has been criticised as being neither practical nor user friendly. Focusing on the allocation of care across different care settings, Lewinter (2004) argues that larger care packages are being awarded to persons in assisted living dwellings, while people living in their own home are increasingly being awarded smaller care packages.

Common Language: Standardising the Home Care Assessment

In the late 1990s an attempt was made at national level to create a system that would improve quality control mechanisms and simplify the task of comparing domiciliary care services across municipalities. With a view to encouraging the use of information technology and documenting domiciliary care provision, a tool called 'common language' (*Foelles sprog*) was introduced. Common language was intended to create a national system whereby the municipalities could award benefits to older people according to need, which would be determined in more or less the same way. It was anticipated that a common terminology would be used by all of the municipalities and that data on care tasks and time awarded to recipients would be collected in a systematic and uniform manner (Csonka and Boll, 2000). However, implementation of common language has been limited, with most municipalities adopting only elements of it. Common language was critisised for being too restrictive (for example, the specification that two and a half minutes could be awarded for brushing teeth). It was also criticised for going against the fundamental principle of domiciliary care in Denmark, which is to enable older people to take care of themselves. The failure of many municipalities to embrace the common language tool has meant that the anticipated comparison and uniformity between the municipalities has been limited.

Despite the failure of the municipalities to adopt the common language tool, national statistics on the Danish home care system are fairly comprehensive when compared with other developed countries. Figures from Statistics Denmark illustrate that the majority of care recipients receive help with both personal care and practical domestic tasks. In 2006, of a total of 206,886 persons who received permanent, continuous home care in Denmark, almost half (49 per cent or 101,181 persons) received both personal and practical care. Forty-one per cent (or 84,989 persons) received only practical care, while 10 per cent (20,716) received only personal care.[5] In 2006 the majority of home care recipients, 56 per cent (116,737 persons) received less than two hours weekly, 12 per cent (24,282) received between 2 and 3.9 hours weekly, 11 per cent (23,327) received between 4 and 7.9 hours weekly, while the remaining 21 per cent (42,540 persons) received eight or more hours home care weekly (Figure 3.2) (Statistics Denmark).

Figures relating to the allocation of hours to all persons aged 65 years and over in 2006 reveal that overall, those aged 80 years or over are awarded more hours of care than those aged between 65 and 79 years. For example, almost 8 per cent of home care recipients aged 80 and over received between 4 to 7.9 hours home care versus just 4 per cent of recipients aged between 65 and 79;

similarly while almost 6 per cent of recipients aged 80 and over received more than 20 hours home care, only 2 per cent of recipients aged between 65 and 79 received such large amounts of home care (Figure 3.3). While these figures reflect the strong home care emphasis in Danish policy they are calculated with 'considerable uncertainty' (Statistics Denmark), and it is unclear if they include care awarded in assisted living dwellings.

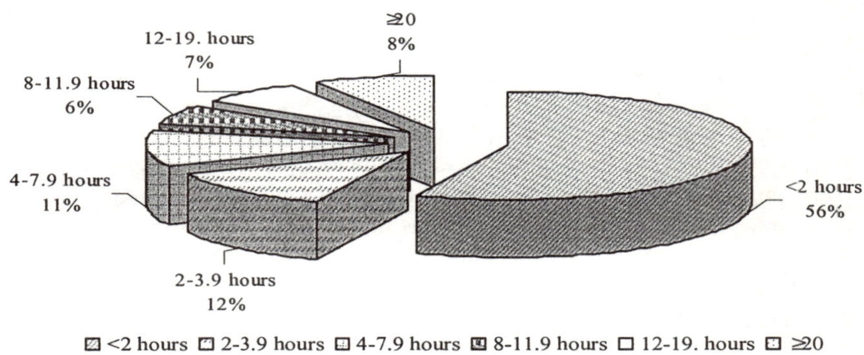

Source: Statistics Denmark.

Figure 3.2 Number of hours per week of home care received by Danish home care recipients, 2006

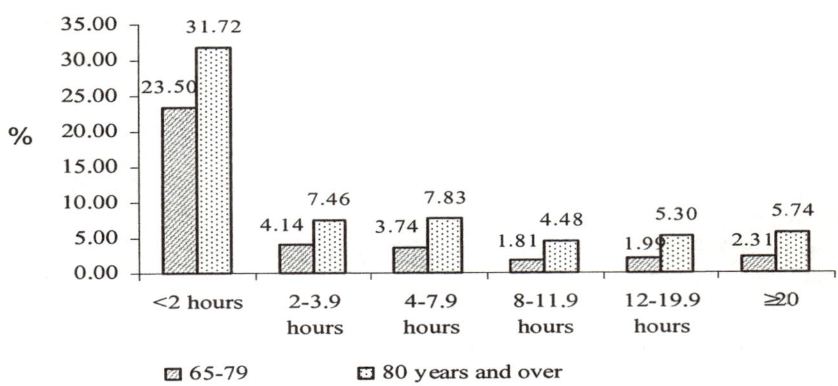

Source: Authors' own calculations based on figures supplied by Statistics Denmark.

Figure 3.3 Number of hours per week of home care received by persons aged 65-79 years, compared with persons aged 80 years and over

Preventive Home Care Visits

The older population of Denmark is systematically screened for care needs: the approach to identifying and assessing care needs is, therefore, very proactive. As Jarden and Jarden (2002) assert, care is brought *to* the person, instead of the person seeking out care. As a result of the 'Roedovre project' in 1984 (Hendriksen et al., 1984), which illustrated the beneficial effects of prevention of illness and psychological problems, a new law entitled 'Preventive Home Visits to the Ageing' was passed in 1998. Since then, each municipality is obliged to pay a preventive home visit at least twice a year to people aged 75 years or over. As well as removing any stigma attached to the notion of domiciliary care, these visits ensure that contact with the older person has, in most instances, begun before a problem has emerged (Rostgaard and Fridberg, 1998). Commenting on the purpose of these visits, a Ministry of Social Affairs (2002, p. 46) report states:

> [T]he aim of the home call service is to create a sense of security and well-being and also to give advice and guidance about activities and support services (both private and public). Another objective is to support elderly people in putting their personal resources to better use and maintaining their functional capacity for as long as possible.

The older person can also decide 'what subject should be discussed during the call' (ibid., p. 46). Irrespective of whether care is deemed necessary, the public health nurse continues to visit annually to re-evaluate the individual's care needs and to follow up any grievances that the domiciliary care recipient may have about the service. A three-year controlled feasibility study on the value of preventive home care visits found that regular visiting was associated with better functional ability, particularly among the oldest group (that is, 80 plus) (Hendriksen and Vass, 2005).

Quite a large proportion of the population of older people refuse the offer of a preventive home care visit, which perhaps reflects the fact that the majority of older people do not require formal home care assistance. None the less, as illustrated in Table 2.1, more than half of Danish citizens aged over 75 years of age do accept the offer and request a preventive home care visit (Statistics Denmark).[6]

Table 3.1 Number of persons who accepted or refused a preventive home care visit by age, 2005

Age	Number who refused a home visit	Number who accepted one or more home visits
75–79 years	60,360	55,986
80–84 years	41,434	49,375
85+ years	24,333	38,321
Total	126,127	143,682

Source: Statistics Denmark (www.dst.dk/HomeUK.aspx).

Quality Control

The Danish home care system is contractualised and rights based (Sjørup, 2004). If the recipient is not satisfied with the service, there are institutionalised procedures for making complaints (ibid.). Regulation and inspection of domiciliary care is conducted at both local and national levels. All local authorities have a senior citizens' council[7] and a Social Board of Appeal to which grievances relating to the home care services can be directed (Ministry of Social Affairs, 2002). At a national level, complaints can by made to one of the seven *Tilysn*, which are independent of the municipality. In extreme instances, grievances can be brought to a national board, under the auspices of the Ministry of Social Affairs, which will assess the adequacy of the service and its compliance with the law. The newly created post of ombudsman, a complaints channel that is unique to Copenhagen, was established to help citizens there to formulate complaints.

In 1998 the Minister for Social Affairs mandated local authorities to draw up a formal policy of quality standards for personal care to cover service agreements, access to service, forms of service provision, policy on working conditions, occupational health and absence of employees through sickness. However, according to interviewees, in recent years much of the emphasis on domiciliary care has been on the remodelling of the new domiciliary care system and the reshuffling of the duties of municipalities. The issue of quality is only recently beginning to emerge as a priority on the domiciliary care agenda. An interviewee in the Ministry of Social Affairs spoke about this new focus as follows:

> We have in recent years focused on the framework and now we are focusing more and more on the quality. Our minister has just put forward a project on quality in the elder sector and we are going to have national workshops and conferences to discuss what is quality, and we will involve families, older people, researchers, municipality officials and politicians to discuss what quality means

> and how to develop quality standards, what expectations we have and what barriers there are. (Interviewee in the Ministry of Social Affairs)

FINANCING STRUCTURE

Home care is financed through state, county and municipal taxes. Redistribution or financial equalisation of taxes is practised to compensate for regional diversity in tax revenue and population structure (Vallgårda et al., 2001). A range of factors are considered for this redistribution process, including age distribution, the proportion of single older people, unemployment levels, the number of persons living in socially deprived areas, the number of immigrants and the number of people in the area who are uneducated (ibid.). According to Vallgårda et al. (2001), expenditure on care for older people rose from 7,733 million Danish krone (€10,376 million) in 1980 to 18,671 million Danish krone (€25 million) in 1999. Nevertheless, Denmark has made considerable fiscal savings by shifting the emphasis away from nursing home care and towards community care. Merlis (2000) calculates that the country's efforts to move from institutional care to care in the community resulted in a drop of spending from 2.6 per cent of GDP in 1982 to 2.3 per cent in 1994 (see Chapter 2 for further figures on social care spending as a proportion of GDP in Denmark).

DELIVERY STRUCTURE

While municipalities are free to avail themselves of public and private providers for services, the tradition of public provision still prevails at this rather early stage following the introduction of 'Freedom of Choice for the Provider' in 2003. Although the majority of municipalities have two or three private providers operating alongside the public provider, in a small number of municipalities there are still only public providers. According to a number of interviewees, however, the monopoly of the public provider is altering, particularly in urban areas, in favour of a greater provider mix. According to interviewees the shift to a plurality of providers has brought some challenges. Private providers have voiced grievances about the unequal playing field in which they and the public providers compete. For instance, the former argue that the costs of insuring staff, purchasing cars and transport are not factored into the price offered by the municipality. Public providers, on the other hand, are able to factor such costs into their generic budget, which consequently does not influence the cost of their service. Therefore it is possible that cost restrictions placed at the municipal level could inhibit the growth of the market and fail to attract new market players.

Currently the remit of the private providers is narrower than that of the public suppliers: typically, the private providers offer help with cleaning and shopping rather than personal care. According to Statistics Denmark, in 2006 there were a total of 600 private suppliers in Denmark, although these providers do not all necessarily deliver care via public funds. Rostgaard (2004) notes that 63 per cent of municipalities have a purchaser–provider model where the older person can choose among more than one provider for practical assistance, 41 per cent offer more than one provider for personal care, and 15 per cent offer more than one provider for meals-on-wheels. In addition, Rostgaard comments that private domiciliary care is predominantly available in the more urbanised areas and is usually accessed by new domiciliary care recipients. Overall, 2 per cent of home care recipients accessed personal care services from the private sector, 22 per cent accessed help for practical assistance (such as domestic help) and 16 per cent of beneficiaries accessed meals-on-wheels services from a private provider. A number of persons interviewed believed that private providers have an advantage over their public counterparts when trying to attract new customers. For example, the former can offer supplementary services such as accompanying a person to the supermarket in return for an additional fee. This is not possible through the public mode. Furthermore, most of the private providers guarantee that the same carer will be allocated to the client, an issue that was found to be problematic in the public sector, with many care recipients complaining of a lack of continuity with respect to the public care worker.

Issues Relating to the Care Workforce

The domiciliary care sector in Denmark is dominated by women. The workforce is largely unionised, with more than 80 per cent of domiciliary carers belonging to a trade union. FOA represents paraprofessional care and health workers, who account for 100,000 of its 180,000 members. It has been active in discussions about the use of private firms to provide care, issues relating to training, delivery of quality care as well as the image of the home care sector as a whole.

The majority of carers are engaged as part-time employees, working approximately 30 hours per week. According to FOA, the average age of a domiciliary care worker is 47 years. Their average gross monthly salary is approximately €2,500, with workers in the private sector being able to command a somewhat higher salary. According to anecdotal reports from an official in FOA, many carers combine work in the private and public sectors. An attractive feature of the private sector is the increased flexibility and control of working time that it allows. Moreover, the salary of carers in the private sector is closely related to their training qualifications, with those with nursing qualifications commanding the highest salary.

The home care workforce is a relatively skilled sector in comparison with other countries. Each municipality decides the level of education and qualifications that are necessary for domiciliary care staff. Korczyk (2004) comments that Denmark has recognised the importance of professionalising care work and enabling career progression within the sector. As of 1998, 48 per cent of domiciliary care staff were social and health assistants who had received one year of training consisting of practical work and some theory, 23 per cent were trained nursing aides, while 10 per cent had no formal education (Rostgaard and Fridberg, 1998). The number of both social and health service helpers and assistants who completed training grew by nearly 11 per cent between 1995 and 1998 (Jensen and Hansen, 2002). In an effort to entice more workers into the domiciliary care field, the municipality of Copenhagen has initiated training programmes that pay the prospective carer a full salary while undertaking training for up to three years; places within this scheme, however, are limited and specific age criteria have to be satisfied.

Nonetheless, among those interviewed, there was unanimous agreement that employment in the home care sector is generally not viewed as attractive and that this perception can negatively influence recruitment and retention of workers. To better understand issues relating to the care workforce FOA (2005) examined conditions that influence the quality of domiciliary care work as well as employee retention. It found that home care workers who had least autonomy in their work and who considered that they were not able to provide the best care felt most negatively about their work and workplace. According to the domiciliary care workers FOA interviewed, strict time monitoring and control have negative effects on their work, jeopardising the quality of care delivered and decreasing work satisfaction. Furthermore, salary, adverse work conditions and poor management were found to influence a carer's decision to leave the home care sector.

FOA estimates that a further 6,500 domiciliary carers will be required in the next ten years. However, in some parts of Denmark recruitment difficulties have already been experienced. According to a number of interviewees, due to recruitment difficulties stipulations on training requirements have been compromised. For example, during the summer months a shortage in the supply of care workers in some areas has led to the recruitment of students – a cohort that has been criticised as being a largely unskilled and transient group of workers. In addition, some municipalities also use the public domiciliary care sector for the purpose of activating social assistance recipients (who are required to take up a work placement in order to fulfil benefit entitlement and re-entitlement criteria). It is possible that the 'forced' employment of these workers may lead to a greater belief that domiciliary carers do not require specialist training or qualifications. With the introduction of publicly purchased private home care, pre-specified costs for care and practices such as the employment of social welfare recipients in the domiciliary care sector, a decrease in training levels, at least for some home care workers, may be inevitable.

Informal Care

The Danish social care system places neither practical nor financial responsibility for the long-term care needs of an ageing relative on family members. Indeed, the European Observatory on Ageing and Older People states that Denmark is alone among the EU member states in not placing the bulk of the responsibility for care on families (Kröger, 2001). Notwithstanding this, the Danish domiciliary system does not actively discourage informal carers from providing care within the formal care system. Rather under the social care system there are specific guidelines for incorporating informal carers, so that a domiciliary care recipient is allowed to employ a family member or neighbour as a carer. In general, they can assist with practical domiciliary care tasks such as cleaning and shopping, although they are not permitted to deliver personal care unless they have the relevant qualifications. The municipality, which acts as the employer, must first approve the person. The carer is paid the same rate of pay as a public domiciliary carer and is covered by the same working conditions. The option of employing an informal carer, however, is not often taken up. As one commentator explained, the culture of public provision is so strong that the majority of care recipients do not view this alternative as an attractive option:

> Most of the elderly I have spoken with, every time we raised the issue of informal care and whether relatives should help out it was totally refused. And it's not something that surprised me because this is something we expect the public sector to take care of. (Interview with academic/researcher)

Such sentiments are in marked contrast to views in countries such as Germany (Chapter 5) and, to some extent, the United States (Chapter 4) where close relatives are widely expected to have extensive responsibilities towards older family members, in terms of either providing a large part of the care themselves, or financing such care if carried out by outsiders. It seems clear that, in combination with other major social and economic characteristics such as female employment rates, the existing structure of social care provision in Denmark acts as a powerful influence on perceptions of the proper remit of public and private responsibility.

Undoubtedly, care is provided by family members and relatives although this is usually of a supplementary nature and provided in conjunction with formal care services. Research has indicated that while only a small minority of persons over 70 years of age live with their children, a large proportion receive some form of help from relatives, friends or neighbours (Stuart and Weinrich, 2001). Help received from children is mainly for practical tasks such as laundry or minor household repairs (Rostgaard and Fridberg, 1998). Formal and informal help seem to complement each other, so that older people with most help from family and friends are also most likely to receive public domiciliary care (ibid.). A study by Holstein et al. (1997) showed a division of labour between informal and formal domiciliary carers. Informal carers were found to provide help with more episodic activities (for example, gardening, repairs and economic advice) and were less involved in daily activities such as cleaning and cooking, which were more frequently perceived to be the responsibility of the home care assistant.

It is possible that the care infrastructure may change in the coming decades and that the third sector (that is, the family) may become an increasingly important player in the provision of care services. Drawing parallels between recent developments in Sweden, Lewinter (2004) points out that the recent rationing of care services in Denmark has meant that care recipients will need to obtain additional services either from family members or from private home care providers. The first option is more likely to be applicable to lower-income marginalised groups while the better-off middle classes will more likely be able to purchase supplementary care. Lewinter argues that current statistics on the provision of home care (which include delivery of intensive care packages in assisted living complexes) currently mask such care arrangements.

CONSUMER POWER

Consumer power in Denmark has increased substantially since the 'Greater Choice for the Provider' legislation in 2003 introduced the concept of 'free choice'. 'Free choice' is very much the cornerstone of the liberal conservative government, which came to power in 2001. It essentially accords domiciliary care recipients greater power to dictate the type of service they receive and thus introduced an element of flexibility not previously present in the Danish system.

The 'Greater Choice for the Provider' legislation, which introduced a purchaser–provider split, increased the consumer *choice* of domiciliary care recipients since it enabled them to choose a public or for-profit care provider. In addition, consumer *direction* was further consolidated with the 2003 legislation. For the first time, a care recipient was legally authorised to ask a domiciliary carer to conduct a different task from what had been specified by the home care assessor. There are constraints as to what tasks the carer is obliged to do and the carer has the right to refuse to do a task if she/he knows that the client has more pressing care needs. One interviewee in the Ministry of Social Affairs spoke of this in terms of a 'negotiation process' that takes place in the home:

> The domiciliary carer has the final word in relation to flexible home care, they have to ask themselves 'is this responsible?', they have to ensure [that] the individual gets what [s/he] needs, the carer can't skip preparing them food or giving them medicine or cleaning the person for long, as that's not responsible, so it's something they have to negotiate with the older person. (Interviewee in the Ministry of Social Affairs)

Free choice is a new concept in the Danish system, and there is an element of cultural change from the perspective of both the care recipient and the carer that has yet to take place. According to interviewees in the Ministry of Social Affairs, preliminary results of a national survey that was recently commissioned found that only 70 per cent of older persons were aware of free choice. Of those who knew about it, 45 per cent had exercised it. A lack of awareness or understanding of the concept of free choice is thus perhaps one of the main reasons for the small number of people using this option. Schultz-Larsen (2004) found that 31 out of 36 municipalities they researched had informed their clients about the availability of flexible domiciliary care, 27 of these did so in writing, while five did not give any information on flexible domiciliary care. Some 22 municipalities informed clients about the right to choose a caregiver, 21 of which did so in writing, while 14 others did not inform their clients about this right at all.

The issue of personal budgets is beginning to be explored at the national level, although at the time of writing this has not yet become a universal entitlement. While Denmark has tended to favour direct service provision over cash-for-care schemes, some municipalities are currently conducting small pilot studies to examine the feasibility of personal budgets. In seven municipalities the elderly are given the opportunity to decide who will provide the care, when it takes place and how. According to interviewees in the Ministry of Social Affairs, early analysis shows that, to date, personal budgets are more appealing to older people in better health and with better functional capacity.

The consequences of increased consumer power are yet to become manifest. The opening of the domiciliary care market to private providers introduces new market dynamics, which is expected to increase competition and, in turn, ensure more efficient delivery of services. Such dynamics should translate into better-quality care for domiciliary care recipients. While the number of private providers operating across the county is currently small, it seems highly probable that private providers will proliferate in the coming years. Rostgaard (2004) offers a useful summary on the introduction of free choice in the Danish context, suggesting that while the choice paradigm confers more 'power' to the care recipient it also transfers responsibility from the municipality to the person in receipt of care. According to Rostgaard (p. 13) the 'freedom to choose includes the risk of choosing poorly, or choosing too often, and thus becoming a bad risk'.

CONCLUSIONS

A number of key legislative changes which have occurred over the past 30 years have ensured that high priority is given to the universal supply of domiciliary care services across Denmark. Access to home care is a universal right and is based on individual care requirements and not on economic circumstances. In short, Denmark provides free care to all older persons who require it, a policy position and reality that appears impossible from the perspective of many other social care regimes where such universal provision is considered both undesirable and excessively expensive.

Providing a comprehensive universal system of care brings with it a number of challenges. At present, seemingly contradictory debates are under way with regard to improving quality of services, on the one hand, and expanding the care workforce to a wider group of unskilled workers, on the other. Financial pressure over the past few years has been reflected in a reduction in the number of hours of care awarded and, in some areas, there has been an increase in the 'targeting' of care to higher-dependency clients and/or a reduction in the provision of domestic care. Already there seem to be some indications that this reduction in care is having negative effects on the quality of care received. What implications this will have on the general public's satisfaction with the welfare state, on levels of informal care and purchase of supplementary private care is something that will become more apparent in the coming years.

In recent years there has been an increasing trend towards a more centralised and uniform regulatory system within Denmark's long-term care system, with an increasing emphasis being placed on quality control and cost documentation. 'The Greater Choice for the Provider' legislation introduced in 2003 refined the duties of municipal administrators and separated the service delivery function from the service monitoring function of municipalities. This has resulted in a new trend of subcontracting care out to private providers. While this legislation has in effect introduced the concept of quasi-markets to the home care system, in reality the public sector is still the dominant supplier of domiciliary care. Population projections estimate that 24.1 per cent of the Danish population will be over 65 years of age in 2040 (OECD, 2006). With such changing demographics, Denmark's ability to offer universal free care will be tested.

NOTES

1. Note, however, that in Denmark the definition of home care includes care delivered in assisted/sheltered housing, which resembles to varying degrees a 'genuine' home setting (Lewinter, 2004).

2. Residents in nursing homes pay for electricity, heating and rent as well as any additional services that they use (Meijer et al., 2000).

3. Since January 2007 Denmark has been divided into 99 municipalities.

4. 'Lov om Social Service nr. 755 af 9. september 2002' granted free choice in relation to domestic care and 'Lov nr. 399 af 6. juni 2002 Frit valg af leverandør af personlig og praktisk hjælp' granted free choice in relation to personal care (Rostgaard, 2004).

5. Authors' own calculations based on figures supplied by Danish Statistics, available at www.statistikbanken.dk/statbank5a/default.asp?w=1024.

6. www.dst.dk/HomeUK.aspx.

7. A report by the Ministry of Social Affairs (2002) notes that these councils are composed of members who have been elected by older persons (persons over the age of 60) in the community. It states that 'the senior citizens' council is to advise the local council in matters of ageing policy, and the council must be consulted about all proposals concerning the elderly' (p. 48).

4. Formal Domiciliary Care in the United States

The welfare and social care system of the United States is characterised by a low provision of public social care services. It is often defined as a liberal regime, meaning that social services are means-tested and the state actively encourages market welfare and services provision (O'Brien and Penna, 1998). In the absence of a protective 'care net', one would assume that the market for private long-term care insurance would be substantial, yet research has shown that less than 6 per cent of US citizens over the age of 45 years have purchased such insurance (Campbell and Morgan, 2005). This would suggest that a large proportion of the US population have no formal protection if the need for long-term care arises.

Wide variations exist between the policies and practical arrangements for long-term care of older people across the different states. While a number of rules govern access to compensatory cash payments obtainable via Medicare and Medicaid, the structures of provision and policy programmes in operation across the states are far from uniform. In this chapter, the focus is on the State of California, and, in particular, a long-term care programme called the In-Home Supportive Services (IHSS) that operates within this state. This programme was chosen because it is by now well established and its coverage extends to a very significant number of people. As such, it provides a good example of an extensive domiciliary care programme in the context of a liberal social care (and welfare) regime. While the bulk of the discussion relates to the IHSS programme at a broader state level, some of it relates to the programme as it functions in the County of San Francisco, reflecting the fact that this is where the majority of fact-finding interviews were conducted.

Before embarking on a discussion of the regulatory, financial and delivery structure of the IHSS programme, this chapter begins by briefly exploring the broader issue of domiciliary care provision within the United States. To understand the domiciliary care system as it relates to California, it is first necessary to have at least a rudimentary understanding of the fundamental structure of the Medicaid system as it now functions. For this reason, a brief introduction to Medicaid and the three types of community care programmes available through it is provided.

THE SHIFT TOWARDS DOMICILIARY CARE

In recent years, there has been an obligation placed on states to provide adequate levels of community care. By law, federal, state and local governments must cater for people with disabilities and older people in a manner that supports self-sufficiency, inclusion and independence. This legal requirement was the result of a 1999 landmark interpretation of Title II of the Americans with Disabilities Act dubbed the 'Olmstead Supreme Court Decision' (Cox, 2005). The *Olmstead* v *L.C.* decision concluded that individuals could not be discriminated against solely on the grounds of disability and that such individuals should be cared for in community rather than institutional settings, where this is deemed appropriate. The implications of this decision were and still are far-reaching. In essence, the federal government specified that each individual state and county is required to do everything in their power to enable people to live in the community. As well as providing a legal justification for de-institutionalisation, the decision also means that services have to be made available in the community to ensure that people who wish to remain living at home have the necessary community resources available to them.

While the federal government has been encouraging states to rebalance their systems to ensure a greater emphasis on home- and community-based services (HCBS), this is still largely at the discretion of each state, and large disparities persist in long-term care systems as well as in the emphasis placed on de-institutionalisation and domiciliary care across the various states. Some states are more advanced than others in this respect. While some states still invest primarily in nursing home care (for example, Mississippi) and have not built up their domiciliary care capacity, others have made greater strides (for example, Oregon). In the United States as a whole, however, spending on institutional care exceeds spending on domiciliary care (see Chapter 2). The dominance of the institutional care sector and growth of large nursing home corporations can largely be attributed to the political lobbying power of the nursing home industry (Kitchener and Harrington, 2004). Allocation of specific government funding through Medicaid funds however, has shifted the balance somewhat towards a greater emphasis on home and community care services (ibid.).

MEDICAID

Public financing of long-term care takes place through two main programmes: Medicaid and Medicare. Medicare is a national social insurance programme paid at 2.9 per cent of annual income split equally between the employee and employer, with no upper limit to the tax base (Karlsson et al., 2004). It is designed to pay only for skilled nursing services that are medically prescribed or home health care.

Medicaid, in contrast, is a tax-funded programme. It was first enacted in 1965 as a joint federal–state entitlement. Medicaid services are means-tested and are available only to those on low incomes. Categories of people covered by Medicaid include older people and people with disabilities. While each of the states regulates its own Medicaid programme, the federal Medicaid statute outlines certain criteria to which states must comply. The US Department of Health and Human Services (2000, p. 8) explains the fundamentals of this legislation:

> The Federal Medicaid statute requires states to specify the amount, duration, and scope of each service they provide, which must be sufficient to reasonably achieve its purposes. States may not place limits on services or arbitrarily deny or reduce coverage of required services solely because of diagnosis, type of illness or condition. Generally, a state plan must be in effect throughout an entire state.

There are three types of Medicaid community care programmes: (i) the home health programme; (ii) the waiver programme and (iii) the state-plan personal care programme. Allocation of finances to each of these is largely left to the discretion of individual states.

First, home health, which states are obliged to provide, was authorised in 1970 and provides services for a short period to individuals with acute care needs. It includes a domiciliary care component. Federal regulations require that home health services include home health aides, nurses, medical supplies and equipment and appliances suitable for use in the home (US Department of Health and Human Services, 2000). However, domiciliary care is available only if skilled nursing services are required and typically lasts for a period of four to six weeks. Of the three community care programmes, this is the only one where annual expenditure is decreasing, which is ironic given that it is the only community care programme that states are obliged to provide.

Second, the waiver programme, was created in 1981. Section 1915(c) of the Social Security Act enables states to request a waiver of certain federal Medicaid requirements and to establish community-based 'waiver' programmes. Under these programmes, states can decide whom and how many people they serve and can run a number of them simultaneously. A cost-control feature (referred to as 'cost neutrality') dictates that participants on the programme cannot have more money spent on them than they would receive if they were in an institution. There has been an expansion of these programmes across the United States in recent years: whereas five years ago only six states ran such programmes, all states, apart from Washington DC, now have at least one, targeted at older people or people with disabilities. Nationwide, there are approximately 250 waiver programmes, with almost a million participants at an annual expenditure of approximately US$18 billion (see Kitchener et al., 2004 for further discussion).

Third, the state-plan personal care programme has been available since the mid-1970s. Currently, these programmes operate in 32 states. The Medicaid state-plan personal care programme grants a great deal of discretion to state officials in relation to the choice of programmes that they run and the eligibility criteria. Generally speaking, the eligibility criteria are more generous or more loosely defined than they are for the waivers. Kitchener et al. (2004) who conducted a national survey of waiver programmes (response rate 76 per cent) found that 57 per cent of them used some sort of financial cap, while 33 per cent used more restrictive financial eligibility criteria than those used for access to institutional services.

IN-HOME SUPPORTIVE SERVICES, CALIFORNIA

The emphasis on home care in California is strong. In the United States, for every two people living in a nursing home facility, one person receives care in the home (Howes, 2005). In California, however, this ratio is reversed: for every three domiciliary care recipients, there is one nursing home care resident (ibid.). In 2002 almost 300,000 people received care though the IHSS state-plan programme. In contrast, just over 70,000 people received care as part of the home health programme, while over close to 60,000 received care through a discretionary waiver programme (Kitchener et al., 2002) (Table 4.1).

Table 4.1 California Medicaid HCBS participants by programme, 2002

	Number of Californian participants	Californian participants per 1,000 population	US participants per 1,000 population
Home health	70,666	2.02	2.57
Personal care services	283,750	8.11	2.01
1915(c) HCBS waivers	59,972	1.71	2.96
Total Medicaid HCBS	414,388	11.84	7.54

Source: Kitchener et al. (2002, Table 1), http://pascenter.org/medicaid/.

Services in the IHSS can be delivered through either an agency contract or an independent provider (IP) contract. Care delivered via the agency contract is subcontracted out to one or more not-for-profit or for-profit agencies that have full responsibility and liability for the care workers they dispatch to IHSS care recipients. Under the IP contract, the home care recipient hires and supervises an individual care worker, whom they have chosen either through their own informal contacts or through formal means, such as a public authority (PA) (see below). While some counties (approximately one-fifth) in the State of California offer services through both contracts, the majority of counties offer only the IP contract. In counties that offer services through both types, people who are socially isolated and are predicted to have difficulty managing and supervising a care worker are usually provided care under the agency contract. Figure 4.1 below offers a visual summary of the two basic structures within the IHSS system.

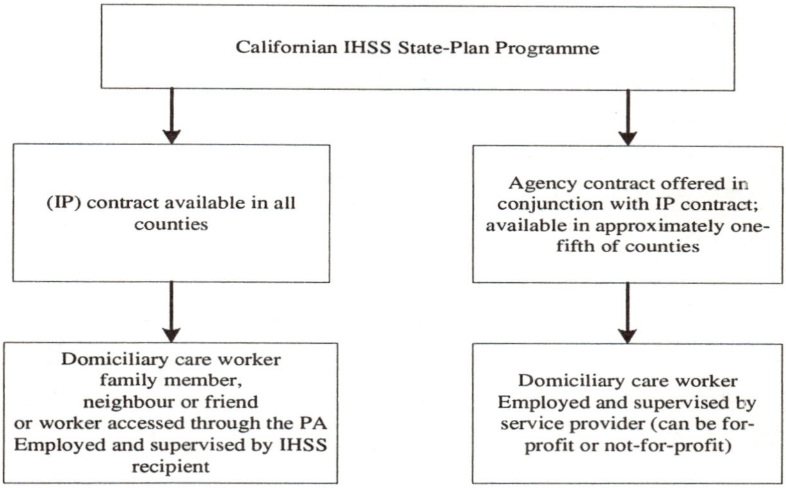

Figure 4.1 The two contracts in the IHSS programme

REGULATORY STRUCTURE

Although the IHSS is a state-run programme, it is administered at county level. While the fundamental structure of the programme is consistent across the 58 counties in California, some administrative differences exist across counties. These differences, which will be expanded upon below, largely relate to the structure of the respective PAs and the availability or absence of an agency contract mode. As mentioned above, the federal government draws up the legislation that permits counties to create their respective state-plan personal care programmes. Decisions regarding the level of services to be offered within this programme are made at state level. The state also finances a percentage of the costs of the programme and has administrative responsibilities, such as processing the payroll of the IHSS workers.

Responsibility of the Department of Health and Human Services

At the county level, the Department of Health and Human Services is granted an element of latitude regarding the delivery of the state-plan personal care programme and the amount of money invested in the programme. The Department is responsible for processing applications for the IHSS; determining financial eligibility of prospective applicants; conducting assessments of the care needs of applicants and routine monitoring of the care awarded through the programme.

Financial eligibility

The first stage in processing applications is for an eligibility assessor to carry out a financial eligibility assessment. Following this, an assessment of functional ability is conducted. Persons on supplementary security income (SSI) or a state supplementary payment (SSP) automatically meet the financial criteria and, hence, do not require a financial eligibility assessment. Financial eligibility is determined at the time of application and reviewed annually or if information about a change in a care recipient's situation is received (California Department of Social Services).[1]

An IHSS care recipient is entitled to possess liquid assets up to a maximum of $2,000, or $3,000 for a couple. All bank accounts are traced back for an 18-month period prior to the submission of the application. Among the items considered as liquid assets are bank accounts, stocks, bonds, cars or recreational vehicles. Ownership of a house occupied by care recipients is not considered when assessing eligibility. Individuals who incur medical and services-related expenses that exceed their income are, in some instances, eligible for IHSS on the condition that they 'spend down' their assets until they have exhausted their ability to pay for the costs of care. In California, the maximum ceiling for liquid assets has not been increased since the mid-1980s. When compared with a number of other states, it can be considered as being quite severe.

Functional status or needs-based assessment

Once financial eligibility has been established, a social worker employed by the Department of Health and Human Services conducts an assessment of the care needs of the applicant. Every prospective recipient receives an in-home assessment that determines levels of physical and cognitive impairment and need for assistance. A social model of need, as opposed to a medical model, informs the IHSS assessment process. It is not based on medical data but rather on how the person's medical problems affect his/her daily functioning. The applicant's physician can complete a form in relation to medication or medical conditions but completion of this form is not mandatory. A standard assessment form called 'uniformit' is used in all 58 counties. The form is used for initial assessments and periodic reassessments of functional capacity. The individual is evaluated on the following activities of daily living and given a ranking of 1 (high functioning) to 5 (low functioning) on each: housework, laundry, shopping and errands, meal preparation, mobility, bathing and grooming, dressing, bowel and bladder, repositioning, eating, respiration, memory, orientation and judgement. When assessing a potential IHSS recipient's care needs, informal care (such as care provided by a spouse) is considered only in relation to domestic chores.

According to interviewees, even though the IHSS is a means-tested entitlement programme, assessment for eligibility can be influenced by the attitudes of county officials, the training of their staff and the gatekeeping enforced in each area. In spite of the existence of a uniform assessment tool, there does seem to be some variability between the counties. For example, San Francisco, a liberal county with a very strong tradition of advocacy in the community, has not capped enrolment and was viewed by some interviewees as being more generous than others in their domiciliary care assessments. These interviewees argued that San Francisco awards more care to people with low levels of dependency than other counties that typically award care only to applicants with high levels of dependency. This means that the county is not targeting services exclusively at people with high levels of dependency but also offers a level of service provision to care recipients with lower levels. Despite variations across counties, the number of people on the IHSS programme has risen, suggesting that there is commitment to the programme in California; state-wide, the average number of IHSS recipients increased by 38 per cent from 1995 (or 190,000 beneficiaries) to 2001 (262,000 beneficiaries) (California Department of Social Services, 2002).

County caseworkers decide whether eligible persons are assigned to an agency or an IP contract. As care subcontracted out under the agency contract mode is substantially more expensive, the majority of care recipients are assigned to the IP contract. Those assigned to the agency contract usually have a cognitive impairment, a psychiatric illness or an addiction problem, and are deemed to be incapable of adequately directing the care worker.

IHSS entitlements are measured in tenths of an hour. Time guidelines for tasks have been identified for particular services, for example, domestic duties may not exceed six hours per month, laundry may not exceed one hour per week (if there are adequate facilities in the home) and food shopping cannot exceed one hour per week. The application must be processed within 30 days following receipt of the application including eligibility determination, the needs assessment and the notice of action. As of October 2005, the average number of hours awarded to IHSS care recipients was 82.5 hours per month. Some 67 per cent of Californian IHSS care recipients are women, half of whom entered the programme as disabled and half as aged. The majority of men (almost 60 per cent) who enter the programme enter as disabled (ibid.).

The Public Authority

The Department of Health and Human Services within each county works closely with a 'public authority'.

A PA is a quasi-governmental agency. It fulfils two functions. First, it acts as 'an employer of record', giving care workers an infrastructure through which to organise, improve job quality, job retention and quality of care. Second, it providers care recipients with a registry of pre-screened care workers. Public authorities were established in the mid-1990s. In 1999, the Californian government passed a law that authorised the creation of 'an employer of record' for the IHSS programme; this could be a PA, a for-profit/not-for-profit organisation or the county itself. The overwhelming majority of counties choose the PA model. The establishment of the PAs ensured lower fiscal spending since it shielded the county from being the employer of the IHSS care workers. If the county acted as the employer, it would then be required to pay the care workers the same pay and social security benefits as other county employees, which would seriously undermine the cost-effectiveness of the programme.

The creation of the PA system served as a successful mechanism to better organise the IHSS domiciliary care workers (working through the IP contract). Prior to their establishment, there was no employer, since the home care workers were considered to be independent care workers (that is, self-employed) by the government. However, as they did not set their own hours or have any say over their pay, terming them independent contractors was a misnomer. Although domiciliary care recipients (or consumer) hired and supervised the care workers, they did not set pay rates or hours of service either. Instead, conditions of employment were determined by the local Department of Health and Human Services and supervised by the state department.

By law, a majority of members making up committees or boards of a PA must be either current or past users of the IHSS. For example, in San Francisco there are 13 representatives on the Board of the Public Authority, comprising seven IHSS care recipients (including older people and people with disabilities), together with representatives from the county commissions, Department of Human Services, Department of Health, Age and Disability Services and a Labour representative who represents the home care workers. The Board has full control over how the San Francisco PA designs its programme and registry.

Quality Assurance

At national level

The Social Security Act mandates the establishment of minimum health and safety standards that must be met by providers and suppliers participating in the home health Medicaid programme. These standards are outlined in the Code of Federal Regulation (CFR) Title 42. Part 484 of the CFR relates specifically to the regulation of home health agencies, delivering care via the home health programme. It requires that home health aides must complete a specific training programme, which addresses a specific range of topics[2] through classroom and supervised training totalling at least 75 hours. At least 16 hours are devoted to supervised practical training and participants must have completed at least 16 hours of classroom training before beginning supervised practical training.

These stipulations do not relate to either state-plan or waiver programmes. Therefore, the federal government places a greater emphasis on the 'inputs' of the home health programme than in either the waiver or state-plan personal care programme. Section 1929 (§1396t) of the Code of Federal Regulation outlines the boundaries within which the states must comply in order to receive grants for home community care programmes for older people with functional disabilities. These boundaries are quite broad and enable the states to enforce and develop their own regulations and quality standards. The national code specifies, however, that the states must develop a standardised assessment instrument to determine eligibility and that each individual identified as being functionally disabled shall be reassessed periodically and no less than once every 12 months. Community care case managers in a not-for-profit or public agency must visit the home care recipient no less than once every 90 days. In addition, the code specifies a number of minimum requirements, which are quite broad but afford some form of protection to the home care recipient. These include 'the right to be fully informed in advance, orally and in writing of the care to be provided . . . and to participate in planning care or changes in care', 'that individuals providing care are competent to provide such care', 'the right [of the home care recipient] to voice grievances with respect to services that are (or fail to be) furnished without discrimination or reprisal', and 'the right to education or training for oneself and for members of one's family or household on the management of care'. Each state is also responsible for certifying the compliance of providers of home and community care and must review the performance of providers periodically. In order to do this, each state is obliged to maintain procedures and adequate staffing levels to investigate complaints of violations. If the state uncovers substandard care practices, it is required to 'make a reasonable effort to notify promptly an immediate family member of each such individual'. In such eventualities, the state 'may terminate the provider's participation under the state-plan programme and may provide in addition for a civil money penalty'.

Within the IHSS programme

Within the IP contract of the IHSS programme, there is a rather distinct method of monitoring and supervision. It is chiefly based on the concept of consumer control and the principle that the domiciliary care recipient (or consumer) has complete authority over the supervision and monitoring of the care worker (or provider). In contrast, under an agency contract, it is the agency that assumes liability for the domiciliary care worker and, consequently, is accountable for the monitoring and supervision of its care workforce.

Formal monitoring of IP workplaces takes place only once a year, by social workers from the Department of Human Services. However, the counties' authority to dictate or influence work practices is severely curtailed under the IHSS programme. Even if a county social worker suspects inadequate work practices, he/she does not have the authority to change the IP care worker unless the care recipient gives consent. There is no mechanism to intervene and replace a care worker. To protect against fraudulence or abuse, the state generates a report that lists care workers who have provided more than 300 hours of care a month. Where neglect or abuse is suspected, the Department of Human Services can call for an independent state hearing. Although they do not legally have the right to question the decision of the care recipient, they can defend their action on moral and ethical grounds.

According to a senior civil servant in the Department of Human Services in San Francisco, the resources of IHSS social workers are currently overstretched and some social workers have caseloads of up to 500 care recipients. In this context, adequate monitoring of care workers can become a difficult task, even if carried out at infrequent intervals (for example, once per year). Attempts are being made at the county level to reduce the caseload of social workers to allow more time to focus on the issue of quality. However, according to one interviewee, even if county social workers were entrusted with more power in the supervision process, monitoring would still take place only once a year. This interviewee was also sceptical about the current system of allocating tasks in tenths of an hour, believing that the more detailed the awarded duties are, the more difficult it becomes to monitor whether these tasks are being completed. An alternative solution is that a certain amount of hours are assigned and the care recipient then decides how much time is spent per task. In reality, this often happens as social workers have limited capacity to enforce time stipulations when they visit the care recipient only once a year. Figure 4.2 offers a visual summary of the specific functions of the various bodies within the IHSS programme (note that, for the majority of counties, the inclusion of the agency contract is not valid).

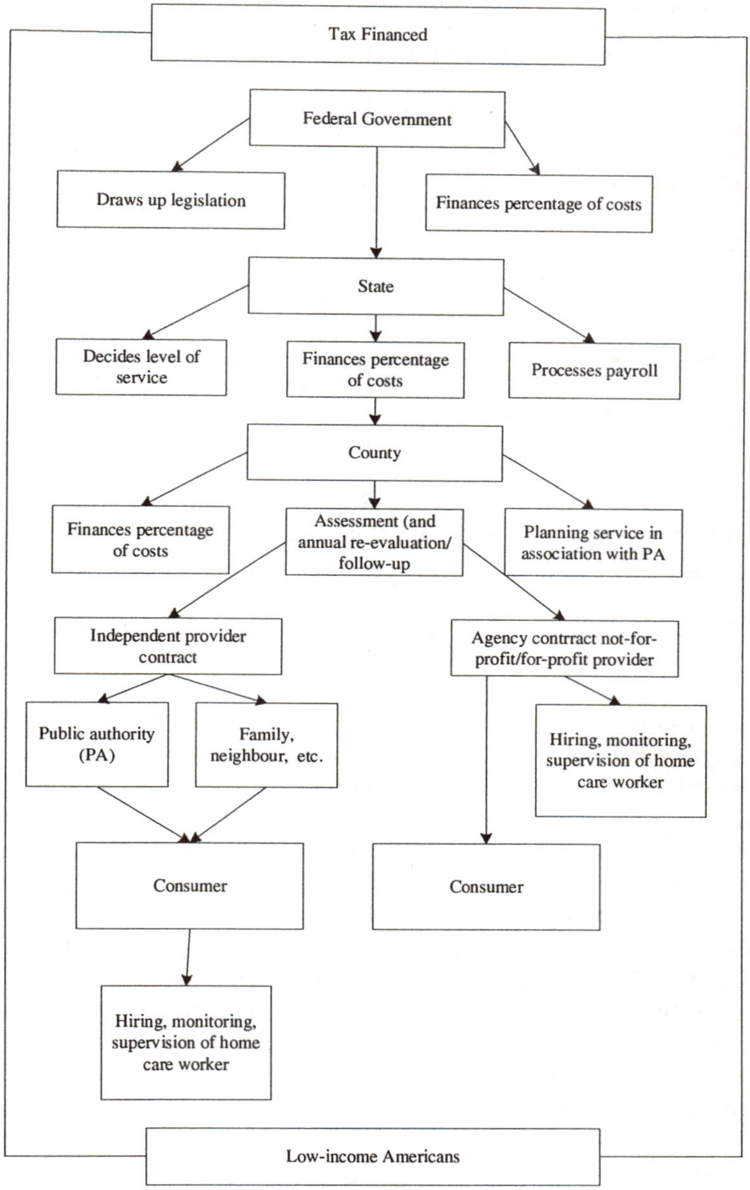

Figure 4.2 IHSS, California

FINANCING STRUCTURE

Total Medicaid spending in the United States for the fiscal year 2004 was $288 billion.[3] Total expenditure on domiciliary nursing care and domiciliary personal care for that year was $46,501 million and $37,623 million, respectively, equating to 46 and 37.3 per cent, respectively, of the overall Medicaid long-term care expenditure.[4] Spending on California's three Medicaid programmes in 2002 is outlined in Table 4.2. The greatest share of funding by far is allocated to the state-plan personal care programme, IHSS, at $1.8 billion in 2001.

Table 4.2 California Medicaid HCBS expenditures, by programme, 2002

	California expenditures	California expenditures per participant	US expenditures per participant
Home health	$578,629,644	$8,188	$3,869
Personal care services	$1,800,000,000	$6,344	$9,177
1915(c) HCBS waivers	$974,812,364	$16,254	$17,126
Total Medicaid HCBS	$3,353,442,008		

Source: Kitchener et al. (2002, Table 1), http://pascenter.org/medicaid/.

As the US Department of Health and Human Services (2000, p. 7) explains, 'states qualify to receive Federal matching funds to help finance [medical] costs by filing a state Medicaid plan document with the Federal Health Care Financing Administration (HCFA)'. Thus, the federal, state and county governments jointly finance the IHSS. The state typically covers 32.5 per cent of the costs, the county 17.5 per cent and the federal government the rest. There are caps on the amount the state and federal government can pay. In California, the state will only cover up to $10.50 an hour for wages and 60 cents an hour for benefits for care workers, while the federal government will only fund up to twice the minimum wage, which is approximately €6.75. While these caps are put on the amount of money the federal and state governments will invest, the county can decide to inject additional funding into the programme. San Francisco and Santa Clare are two counties that have decided to increase the remuneration of care workers beyond the state limit, paying for these additional costs out of their generic budgets. This additional money is channelled to the IHSS care workers to provide them with higher wages and medical and dental insurance.

Due to the considerable growth of the IHSS programme in California and improved wages and benefits secured for IHSS workers, fiscal concerns have been voiced at state level. One implication of this was the abolition of the separate IHSS Residual Programme in 2004. Up to 2004, IHSS services delivered by a spouse were funded through the Residual Programme by California state and county finances. Following concerns about the escalating costs of this programme, the 2004 State Budget called for its termination. A request for a waiver to safeguard the care recipients of this strand of the programme was called for and was successfully granted in August 2004, with a federal waiver programme receiving $1.7 billion in federal funding over five years. As well as safeguarding care recipients in need of protective supervision, it also ensured that the almost 20,000 people receiving care from either a spouse or a parent could continue to do so.

Delivering the vast majority of care via an IP contract as opposed to an agency contract is financially sensible. In San Francisco, for instance, the cost of services from the Consortium (an agency contract) is approximately $22.33 an hour. This contrasts with the approximate sum of $16 an hour that the county pays under an IP contract. For an agency contract provider, overheads such as the employment of human resource personnel, training, monitoring and administrative and supervision staff have to be factored into the pricing structure. While not confirmed in the interviews conducted, it seems likely that the majority of counties do not offer services through the agency contract mode due to the increase in costs it would incur (through, for example, agency and administrative costs and the need for more case workers).

DELIVERY STRUCTURE

The delivery structure of the IHSS programme varies somewhat throughout the 58 counties. The service provider landscape is dependent on whether the county offers services either through an IP contract, or through an IP contract in conjunction with an agency contract. While all states are obliged to provide services via the IP mode, approximately one-fifth of the counties also offer services via the agency contract mode (Benjamin and Matthias, 2004). In addition, variations exist across states in relation to the PA structure as well as wages and entitlements of home care workers, which, undoubtedly, can indirectly affect service delivery. As pointed out above, the IHSS in San Francisco provide services under both the IP and the agency contract modes. As Table 4.3 indicates, almost 16,000 people in San Francisco receive IHSS through the IP mode, while just over 1,000 receive services through the agency contract mode. A further 118 people receive a mix of services through the IP and agency contract modes.

Table 4.3 Breakdown of service delivery mode in San Francisco, 2005

Service delivery mode	Number of persons
IP mode	15,768
Contract mode	1,068
Mixed (IP and contract)	118

Source: Communication from the San Francisco Department of Human Services (November, 2005).

Service Delivery Modes

Independent provider mode

Under the IP mode, the care worker appointed by the IHSS care recipient can be a relative, a friend or a neighbour. The percentage of domiciliary care workers who are family members (versus non-relatives) varies across counties from 29 per cent in Santa Barbara to 81 per cent in Orange County (Daly et al., 2004).

IHSS care recipients can also source a care worker from the PA. Interviewees explained that prior to the establishment of the PA system, there was no coherent recruitment system to help IHSS recipients find a domiciliary care worker. Apart from obtaining names from a few small registries compiled by independent living centres or not-for-profit organisations, most care recipients had to source and screen care workers themselves. The creation of the PA put an end to this, by providing a list of pre-screened care workers. A person interested in working as a home care worker under the IP mode (via the PA), must attend an interview with the PA, a two-hour orientation process, and complete a six-page application form. Once references have been checked, the individual is listed in the PA registry and referred to IHSS care recipients. Largely due to pressure from IHSS care recipients and their advocates, a deliberate decision was taken that the PA would not conduct criminal background checks on care workers. This was based on the fear that the pool of domiciliary care workers would be considerably reduced if they were screened for criminal offences. With recent pay increases for IHSS care workers, it has been argued, however, that the justification behind this argument (that is, a limited pool of available care workers) loses much of its relevance.

The PA has no jurisdiction over IHSS care recipients and has little control over the monitoring of the quality of services delivered in the home. While the PA will record complaints and grievances relating to a domiciliary care worker, it does not take any responsibility for the continuous monitoring of the service. Essentially, if a domiciliary care worker is placed, and no grievances are voiced, the PA will have no further contact with either the care recipient or the care worker. According to interviewees, care workers can generally be fired without notice and without being given a reason. Although it is prohibited to fire a care worker on grounds such as racial, sex or religious discrimination, this can be difficult to prove in the intimate setting of the home. The only employment law that care recipients must adhere to is that if they wish to fire the home care worker, they must furnish him/her with an advance payment of 24 hours' pay.

Agency contract mode

Not all care recipients are able to act as an employer of a domiciliary care worker and, consequently, hire, supervise and manage the care delivered. Those who for health or social reasons cannot are served under the agency contract mode. This option (available in a few Californian counties) is generally only offered to those with serious chronic health conditions.

In the County of San Francisco, all care work provided via the agency contract mode is delivered by a not-for-profit organisation called the Consortium. The Consortium acquired its first contract with the Department of Health Services to provide 150,000 hours in 1994. At the time, it delivered care to IHSS care recipients alongside a for-profit domiciliary care organisation. In 2001, it was awarded the entire contract to provide 850,000 hours of IHSS service. In 2005, the contract was for 730,000 hours serving 1,400 clients. The Consortium provides services to care recipients with the most complex needs in San Francisco's IHSS programme, including those with mental health difficulties, substance abuse problems and multiple chronic conditions. In 2005, 49 per cent of its client base were people aged 65 years and over. However, in an interview a spokesperson for the Consortium pointed out that, increasingly, older IHSS care recipients have to compete with those with mental illness and substance abuse problems to access the Consortium's services. In previous years, up to 80 per cent of their clients were over 60 years of age.

Supervision of the domiciliary care worker engaged under an agency contract is the responsibility of the provider agency with whom the county has entered into a contract. The Consortium in San Francisco requires that care workers have relevant experience of at least one year or evidence of having completed a certified domiciliary care/nursing assistant programme. It offers a 44-hour basic training programme on a monthly basis: although participation is voluntary. Each care worker receives a five-hour orientation before being assigned to a care recipient. Peer mentors assess the 'on-the-job skills' of the care worker during the first two weeks of employment. Where training or skills deficits are identified, additional training is given.

Further assessments are carried out every four months and, thereafter, when a field coordinator meets with a care recipient to observe his or her condition. Follow-up assessments of the care worker are undertaken annually. Punctuality and attendance of care workers is monitored in real-time using SanTrax, a telephony system that enables the care worker to 'sign-in' using the care recipient's home telephone. 'No show' reports are run three times each day. Within the Consortium, supervision is coordinated by three groups: first, service delivery supervisors who match care workers with care recipients; second, field coordinators who perform care recipient assessments quarterly and coordinate ancillary services and, third, peer mentors who provide skills assessments and on-the-job skills training. Each service delivery supervisor is assigned approximately 32 workers to supervise.

Home Care Workers

At a national level

> In general, in many places we find this [care] workforce is ageing themselves. Again, it depends upon the state, but in a lot of places there may be a lot of turnover but there is turnover in the same positions, there are a lot of workers who have been there for a very long time, and then there is a portion that turns over and over again. (Interview with Home Care Workers' Interest Group Representative)

Citing the Bureau of Labor Statistics (2006), the Paraprofessional Health Care Institute (2006) notes that an additional 962,000 direct care positions will be created in the US by the year 2014, resulting in a 41 per cent increase in the number of personal and home care aides. High staff turnover and recruitment difficulties, however, have been experienced in relation to the domiciliary care industry in the United States. Stone (2004, p. 339) notes that, in 2002, 37 states identified worker recruitment and retention as priority issues and believed that further 'demographic and economic trends do not augur well for the future availability of quality domiciliary care workers'.

According to the Paraprofessional Health Care Institute (2006), nine out of ten 'direct care workers' are women. Their average age is 41. Over half are white and non-Hispanic, approximately one-third are African American, while the remainder are from Hispanic and other ethnic minority groups. Two-fifths have a high school diploma or a General Educational Development certificate, while 38 per cent have attended college. A quarter are unmarried and live with children in contrast to 11 per cent of the total working US population. The national annual income for personal and domiciliary care aides in 2005 was $17,710 (ibid.). There is, however, considerable variation across states in relation to the rate of pay for domiciliary care work.

Within the IHSS programme

In California in 2005, there were an estimated 154,322 home and personal care workers, averaging 4.4 per 1,000 persons.[5] Within California, the hourly rate for home care workers in the IP mode varies from county to county. San

Francisco, along with Marin County, offers the highest wage, at $10.50. Prior to the establishment of the PA, wages averaged $4.50 an hour. Anecdotal reports indicate that when wages were this low, many care recipients unofficially reduced the number of hours of care received in an effort to boost the hourly pay and entice more suitable workers.

Workers' compensation benefits or insurance is paid by the state and provided to all care workers. In some counties, social security benefits offered to care workers under the IP mode include health and dental insurance. While agency contract care workers in San Francisco have preferential working conditions (since they receive sick pay, holiday pay and transport costs) compared to workers employed in the IP mode, it would be incorrect to suggest that this is the case for all care workers employed by other agency providers across the State of California. For many care workers employed by other not-for-profit or for-profit organisations, it seems highly probable that social security benefits and security of work contracts are just as precarious as for workers engaged under an IP contract (see Benjamin and Matthias, 2004).

Campaigns by the trade union, the Service Employees' International Union (SEIU), together with the establishment of the PA, were largely responsible for the considerable increase in the rates of pay for care workers. The SEIU has played and continues to play a significant role in the advancement and improvement of the working conditions of and benefits afforded to IHSS care workers. Overall, union membership of domiciliary care workers is high in California. Union dues are charged at 2 per cent of monthly wages, to a minimum of $28 dollars per month. The union offers free training courses to members in areas such as Spanish domiciliary care terminology, and health and safety.

The introduction of higher pay rates and social security benefits has led to an increase in the number of family members engaged as IHSS care workers as well as a stabilisation in the home care workforce. In 1997 the staff turnover rate in San Francisco was 61 per cent; while in 2003 it was approximately 26 per cent (Howes, 2005). As one interviewee noted, 'now we see some of our workers have been working in the system for years'. According to another interviewee, a similar initiative in the state of Wyoming, where wages were raised by over $2 an hour, has also had a dramatic impact on the retention and stabilisation of the workforce.

The issue of home care training has not received much attention within the IHSS programme, perhaps due to the fact that the programme is based on a social model of care as opposed to a medical model. According to interviewees, increased training of care workers has been argued by some in the disability movement to constitute an infringement of the rights of care recipients (as consumers) to dictate the level of training they require from care workers. With an emphasis on the rights of the consumer, the corresponding rights of the employee could potentially be overlooked. In such instances, ironically, models of consumer direction may unwittingly contribute to negative images of the domiciliary care workforce and the belief that it is a low-skilled unprofessional job, and that remuneration does not have to be increased:

> because they are saying I know what I need to live as independently as possible in the community and I don't need a doctor and I don't need a nurse, I need someone who will follow my instructions on how I want to bathed etc. So that's de-professionalising [the care service] in a way, it is like a double-edged sword. (Researcher interviewed at a Californian university)

Within the IP mode, if care recipients are dissatisfied with the work of their care worker, they can reprimand them, reduce their hours and employ an alternative care worker, or alternatively sack them. Such precariousness of the employment contracts of the care workers creates many problems. One interviewee, who works under an agency contract, elaborated upon this and other ergonomic problems by contrasting standards for care workers under an agency contract with standards for those engaged under an IP contract:

> Things like beds being too low and having to lift them out, that happens all the time in IP, here we go in and if we see that, we say, 'no way' and call the Department to get a hospital bed or else forget it, I'm not going to bust the back of a worker. So there are all those health and safety issues that are ignored. And also the whims of the clients means that then the person won't get any money, they can say I'm going away this week, I want to be alone, or my mom is coming I don't need you for two weeks. (Manager in contract agency)

According to an interviewee in the Paraprofessional Health Care Institute, a number of states have made inroads into balancing the competing interests of care workers and care recipients. For example, an experiment in New Hampshire where the independent living centre employs care workers, but allows care recipients to manage their care worker, in terms of dictating the hours of care and so on, seems to have struck a good balance. As part of the contract of service, care recipients are obliged to provide a safe working environment for the care worker, and where this does not happen the independent living centre has the right to terminate care.

CONSUMER POWER

At National Level

In 1999, the Federal Health Care Financing Administration specified:

> [All relatives except] legally responsible relatives (i.e. spouse and parents of minor children) could be paid for providing personal care services . . . and it explicitly recognized that provision of such services may be directed by the people re-

> ceiving them. This consumer direction includes the individual's supervision and training of their personal care attendants. (US Department of Health and Human Services, 2000, p. 12).

Increasingly, states across the US are implementing consumer-directed models of domiciliary care. In the US context, such models give care recipients: (i) the authority to develop their own care service and care plans and (ii) the choice of hiring/firing, scheduling, training, supervising and purchasing services 'and, within the boundaries established by law, directing the payment of the care worker' (ibid., p. 115).

Benjamin (2001) has identified three factors that have stimulated the expansion of consumer-directed programmes in the US: (i) pressure from within the disability movement; (ii) a call for the 'de-medicalisation' of some health conditions and services and (iii) concerns about the cost of long-term care, as well as the fact that consumer direction reduces the need for care agencies and case managers. All but two states in the US offer some sort of consumer-directed long-term care programme, and in total almost half a million people access services from these programmes (OECD, 2005). However, this figure is somewhat deceptive since the majority of these programmes are small, with one-fifth having fewer than 100 care recipients (ibid.). Moreover, the Californian IHSS programme accounts for almost half of all of the estimated participants in consumer-directed programmes in the United States (ibid.).

Within the IHSS Programme

In the State of California, consumer direction is a fundamental aspect of the IHSS programme under both IP and agency contracts. The IP mode, in particular, is a highly consumer-driven model, allowing care recipients to hire, supervise and fire home care workers. The home care recipient not only chooses the care worker but also schedules the work and decides what times the care worker will work and what tasks he/she should complete. The advantages of consumer power within the IHSS programme were commended by all those interviewed. A senior manager in the Department of Human Services, San Francisco, stated:

> Its [the IHSS programme's] greatest asset is that you have control of who is coming into your home, who is bathing you, who is toileting you, you want to feel comfortable with that person. When it gets into personal care you really want to feel comfortable with that person so that's its greatest strength. And for people who can manage it, who can really direct the person and supervise the person, and someone who is not going to be influenced by them, intimidated by the provider, it is a great system. (Interviewee in the Department of Human Services)

Interviewees also regarded as an advantage the fact that consumer power allows a home care recipient to employ a family member, including a spouse or adult child, if they so choose. Allowing the home care recipient to employ a family member in the intimate setting of the home was seen as not only enabling the family unit to stay together but also providing an additional source of income to families that are financially disadvantaged. Another advantage is that consumer-directed models that permit care recipients to employ family members extend the pool of home care workers to a group of workers who may not otherwise enter the home care profession (Stone, 2001). The ability of informal caregivers to work within the IHSS system, also brings with it some possible challenges, for example, does it negatively impact on persons within an ethnic minority and is the care delivered by the care worker in any way compromised due to the fact that in some instances the carer may be juggling care work with formal employment (see Scharlach et al., 2003; Scharlach et al., forthcoming)?

Currently IP contracts under the IHSS consumer-directed system in California provide very few if any supportive services to care recipients, who may need training and assistance in making consumer direction work. Consumers are given an information booklet, which offers suggestions on interviewing domiciliary care workers and monitoring domiciliary care work. However, limited resources mean that none of the agencies – the county, the social workers or the public authority – can give enough time to discussing any grievances or concerns that care recipients may have in this regard.

A number of interviewees pointed out that, in some instances, a consumer-directed system that gives more autonomy and control can disadvantage individuals and families who are already disadvantaged, vulnerable or less capable. As one interviewee phrased it, 'the consumers get to make choices even if they are bad choices'. The IP system, arguably, favours those who have the most resources, cognitively, physically, socially and psychologically, as this cohort is better able to hire and supervise the care provided. An academic working in the area voiced the following concerns:

> [Consumer direction] ultimately allows society to consider long-term care issues as problems of the individual, as opposed to societal problems and it allows . . . society to say 'we are going to cap the number of dollars', 'we're going to say you get x number of dollars and if you can't get the care you need that's your problem' as opposed to having a societal stake in ensuring that people who need care get care so it moves the onus to the individual and away from the welfare state. I see it as one of many efforts to move away from a welfare state approach to a much more individual approach. (Researcher from Californian university)

Some US states have managed better to combine the integration of consumer direction with formal support services than California. For example, Oregon's Medicaid programme allows home care recipients to hire and fire their home care worker, but only with the guidance of a case manager (Benjamin, 2001).

In Maine, specialist training courses on hiring and supervising care workers are offered to care recipients who are deemed to have the ability to self-direct their own care, while in New Hampshire and Utah care recipients with developmental disabilities are granted consumer choice by selecting a support team to help with service delivery decision making (ibid.).

The evidence is inconclusive as to whether all care recipients prefer to be able to hire, fire and supervise their own care workers. Benjamin et al. (2000), found that care recipients under self-directed consumer-directed models consistently report more positive outcomes than those receiving care under an agency contract. Benjamin et al. (1999) also found that home care recipients in the IP mode were at no greater risk of abuse and neglect than recipients in the agency mode. In a separate study, based on interviews with a random sample of 1,095 IHSS care recipients, Benjamin and Matthias (2001) found that while younger home care recipients were more likely to employ someone they know, older recipients were more likely to hire a relative as a carer. Benjamin and Matthias (ibid.) argue that the findings reflect the fact that older people have smaller (and more family-based) support networks than younger people. They concluded that while there are no substantial differences between younger and older IHSS care recipients, older recipients tended to be somewhat less enthusiastic about consumer direction than younger ones, and this difference was viewed as being marginal. An analysis of 731 long-term care recipients by Sciegaj et al. (2004) indicated that older people's preference for consumer direction span a continuum, with some people preferring control over certain aspects of their care. The researchers also found not only that perceptions of consumer direction were different between different racial or ethnic groups but also that there were great differences within groups. They attributed this heterogeneity to other life situational or attitudinal factors, suggesting that interpersonal factors and life experiences can play an important role in a person's perception of consumer direction.

CONCLUSIONS

The main public programme contributing to the financing of domiciliary care services in the United States is the means-tested Medicaid programme. States have considerable latitude in deciding how much emphasis is placed on community versus institutional care, and how much money they want to invest in both. While they must provide home health care, and can apply for waivers, states also have the option of offering state-plan personal care programmes, which receive federal dollars to support the costs. Unlike waivers, state-plan personal care programmes and home health programmes are entitlement means-tested programmes which must be provided if pre-established criteria are set. This means that the potential for costs to escalate is high given demographics projections that predict an ageing of the population.

The IHSS in California is the largest state-plan personal care programme in the United States. While administered at state level, the main responsibility for regulation and delivery of the services lies at county level. Service provided under the IHSS can be delivered via IP or agency contracts. The former model, which is supported by the PA system, entrusts the responsibility of hiring, firing and supervising the care worker to the care recipient. The more controlled agency contract mode is available in only a handful of counties, and delivers care via contracted service providers to a domiciliary care recipient with high care needs who is deemed unable to supervise his/her own care. The availability of both an IP and agency contract is arguable ideal; however, given the higher financial costs of the latter, it is unlikely that additional counties will introduce agency contract services.

Consumer power and the rights of the care recipient have long played an important role in the US domiciliary care system. Under the IHSS, consumer power, as manifested in the IP mode, is a prime example of how far the concept of consumer control can be advanced. There are however a number of unresolved complexities particular to the consumer-directed mode of the IHSS programme. Matters such as specification of minimum training requirements, background checks, employee rights and objective monitoring and supervision are contentious issues, as some interest groups argue that state/county regulation of any kind is an infringement on the rights of the care recipient.

Finally, the recruitment, employment and retention of care workers within the US will become an issue of increasing importance in the coming years. Long-term care programmes that are essentially budget driven could jeopardise the rights of care workers. At a time when numerous national interest groups are lobbying for increased investment in the care workforce, models such as the cash and counselling model, which allows consumers to spend their money as they wish, may have negative consequences for the rights of care workers. The challenge thus lies in protecting care workers, while refraining from infringing on the rights of care recipients to self-direct their care.

NOTES

1. Available at www.cdss.ca.gov/cdssweb/IHSSEligib_174.htm.

2. These include communications skills, observation, reporting and documentation of patient status and the care or service furnished, reading and recording temperature, pulse and respiration, basic infection control procedures, basic elements of body functioning and changes in body function that must be reported to an aide's supervisor, maintenance of a clean, safe and healthy environment, recognising emergencies and knowledge of emergency procedures, the physical, emotional and developmental needs of and ways to work with the populations served

by the Home Health Agency, including the need for respect for the patient, his or her privacy and his or her property, and appropriate and safe techniques in personal hygiene and grooming.

3. This figure includes state and federal expenditures. It includes benefit payments and disproportionate share hospital payments; it does not include administrative costs, accounting adjustments, or the US Territories. Total spending including these additional items was about $296 billion in 2004 (Urban Institute and Kaiser Commission on Medicaid and the Uninsured estimates based on data from Centers for Medicare and Medicaid Services-64 reports, Urban Institute and Kaiser Commission, September 2005).

4. The Kaiser Commission on Medicaid and the Uninsured, available at www.kff.-org/mfs/medicaid.jsp? r1=CA&r2=US&x=10&y=10.

5. Center for Personal Assistance Services calculations based on information obtained from the 2005 American Community Survey. Available at http://pascenter.org/state_based_-stats/acs_workforce_state_2005.php?title=Number%20of%20Home%20and%20Personal%20Care%20Workers&state=california.

5. Formal Domiciliary Care in Germany

Rostgaard and Fridberg (1998, p. 486) characterise Germany as:

> a conservative and corporatist type of welfare state–conservative because the role and responsibilities of the family are stressed in the German welfare state, and corporatist because implementation of the 'social state' is carried out by non-government insurance associations and large associations of independent welfare providing service agencies, within the framework set out by legalisation and public authorities.

Offering a different perspective, Cuellar and Wiener (2000, p. 10) point out that the German welfare system places a strong emphasis on social solidarity and the 'belief that collective arrangements that protect everyone, not just the poor against the exigencies of life (such as sickness, retirement, and disability), are desirable'. Up to the mid-1990s, care for the frail and disabled in Germany was means-tested and the responsibility of the local state governments, the *Länder*. Prior to the introduction of long-term care insurance (LTCI) in 1994, the financing of long-term care took place primarily through private spending and, for those without access to 'free' family care or monetary sources to meet the costs of care, through means-tested social assistance from the local government.

By the late 1980s, increasing numbers of older people requiring long-term care placed inordinate financial pressure on the local governments. For example, over 80 per cent of nursing home residents in West Germany and 100 per cent in East Germany were reliant on means-tested social assistance (Cuellar and Wiener, 2000). As a result of increasing fiscal pressures and issues relating to the inequities of long-term care coverage, policy debates became heated and calls for a universal long-term care insurance programme were advanced. In April 1994, the Social Dependency Insurance Act introduced compulsory, universal social insurance for long-term care (Pfegeversicherung). As a result of this Act, Germany provides extensive universal nursing home and domiciliary care benefits for older people and younger people with disabilities. The clear majority of persons who access long-term care services via the LTCI funds are over 65 years of age: Rothgang (2003) calculated that 78 per cent of all beneficiaries are aged 65 years or older and that over 50 per cent of these are 80 years or over.

Until 1994 there were four social insurance schemes covering the social risks of retirement, sickness, unemployment and industrial accidents. LTCI was, therefore, the fifth 'pillar' in the German social insurance structure. All German citizens are obliged to pay LTCI contributions and depending on their employment status can enter the statutory scheme or choose a private scheme. Irrespective of which scheme they choose, benefits are universal and based on functional ability: the applicant's financial means and family situation are not considered in the assessment. In December 2004, a total of 2.05 million people acquired either domiciliary care or institutional care through the LTCI programme. In total, approximately 1.38 million LTCI beneficiaries acquired domiciliary care, 1,281,398 beneficiaries received these services through the public LTCI funds, while approximately 80,000 accessed services through private LTCI funds (Federal Ministry of Health and Social Security, 2005).

REGULATORY STRUCTURE

Equity and parity of the LTCI programme was emphasised from the outset of the scheme, with legal guidelines and universal eligibility criteria established at national level. The introduction of LTCI saw the local governments lose much of their regulatory authority in the area of long-term care. However, while the LTCI legislation is specified by central government, any amendments to the legislation will generally not take place without the support of the *Länder* and the *Bundesrat* (the upper chamber of the German legislature consisting of representatives of the *Länder*) (Brodsky et al., 2000; Campbell and Morgan, 2005).

The *Länder,* which had previously paid for long-term care through the social assistance system, made considerable cost savings with the introduction of the LTCI scheme (see Bönker and Wollmann, 2005). While they no longer have financial responsibility for long-term care, they still have an obligation to ensure that sufficient provisions are made to deliver long-term care through the insurance funds and that an 'adequate care infrastructure' is in place so that the LTCI programme can function in an optimal manner. To do this, they were instructed to spend half of the savings made from the introduction of the LTCI programme on improving the care infrastructure (Karlsson et al., 2004). The notion of the right infrastructure is a somewhat ambivalent and illusive concept and is open to different interpretations. The law states that the LTCI funds are not responsible for the start-up investment costs of formal service providers, and, instead, delegates this responsibility to the *Länder*. This duty, however, is not enshrined in the law and it seems that some *Länder* have been reluctant to pay for the start-up costs of formal home care providers and do not always provide adequate support to the private service providers (Brodsky et al., 2000). Organisations such as the Senate Administration for Health, Social Affairs and Consumer Protection, which are unique to each *Länder,* inspect the planning and infrastructure that the *Länder* put in place and ensure that the *Länder* are fulfilling their legal obligations within the LTCI programme.

The LTCI programme was not conceived of as a full coverage scheme, and, as a result, either additional informal care or supplementary privately funded care may need to be accessed by the many people whose care needs exceed those covered through LTCI. As a result, private co-payments and means-tested social assistance play an important role for a large proportion of people. Despite this, however, the proportion of LTCI recipients who are eligible for additional social assistance to help fund these costs is negligible (Cuellar and Wiener, 2000). This is not the case for nursing home care, where overall 50 per cent of LTCI nursing home residents are dependent on social assistance. Cuellar and Wiener (p. 12) point out that this is perhaps 'a transition issue that will decline as the institutionalized population that depleted its assets prior to the new program dies off'.

Responsibility of the Insurance Funds

The LTCI funds are the most powerful actors in the regulation of the LTCI programme. In total there are more than 400 insurance funds (Karlsson et al., 2004). These funds are responsible for the implementation of the legal provisions, including the collection of insurance contributions and the payment of benefits, the assessment and eligibility processes, quality assurance (in association with the Medical Office of the Sickness Fund) and the negotiation of contracts with the service providers. The funds are divided into public and private insurance schemes. Criteria for entry and practices of both public and private schemes are highly regulated and bound by many legal obligations which are enforced at the federal level. The highly regulated administrative system governing the LTCI funds means that there is essentially no competition between these funds since both contribution rates and benefits are uniform (Rothgang, 2003). The Senate Administration for Health, Social Affairs and Consumer Protection, which supervises the *Länder*, is also responsible for the legal supervision of both public and private insurance companies. The Senate cannot interfere with any specialist tasks related to the insurance funds, but rather ensures that they are working in accordance with the LTCI legislation. In addition to supervising the *Länder* and the insurance funds, the Senate deals with the complaints and petitions filed by citizens.

Eligibility Assessment

The use of a national universal assessment tool ensures that parity in the eligibility assessment is guaranteed within Germany's LTCI programme. Detailed eligibility criteria are written into law and use of different or additional considerations is forbidden. The eligibility assessment is conducted by medical nurses employed by the Medical Services of the Health Insurance system (Medizinischer Dienst der Krankenversicherung, MDK). Since 1 January 2000, individuals must have been insured for at least five of the ten years preceding the filing of an application.1 The basic criteria for obtaining LTCI benefits is fulfilled when the applicant has limitations in two or more activities of daily living (ADL) and a need for help in some instrumental activities of daily living (IADL). Eligibility is determined through assessment of the duration and frequency of help regularly required with personal hygiene, eating, mobility and housekeeping, and is granted to people who at a minimum require personal care for at least 1.5 hours per day over a six-month period or longer.

Eligibility is measured on the basis of three levels of disability: substantial, severe and very severe, with the different levels of dependency corresponding to maximum expenditure per person at each level. People with *substantial* care needs (care level 1) have limitations in two or more ADL at least once a week and need help with IADL several times a week. Care is classified as being required for a minimum of 90 minutes per day based on the productivity of an average informal care worker (Brodsky et al., 2000). People classified as having *severe* care needs (care level 2) have at least three limitations with ADL and need help with IADL several times per week, in this instance, a minimum of three hours of care is required daily (ibid.). Finally, those classified as having *very severe* care needs (care level 3) have limitations in ADL both day and night and need help with IADL several times a week. People who fall into this category are categorised as requiring more than five hours of assistance on a daily basis (ibid.).

Table 5.1 indicates the percentage breakdown of care recipients by the three care categories as of December 2003. It suggests that the majority of people are awarded services at care level 1, with a slightly greater proportion of beneficiaries covered by the public programme allocated services within this care level (57.5 per cent through the public LTCI funds versus 50.8 per cent through the private LTCI funds). At care levels 2 and 3, there is also a marginal difference between the proportion of care awarded by the private and public insurance funds, with those covered by private insurance funds more frequently allocated to care levels 2 or 3. It is difficult to determine whether this discrepancy is the result of a more 'lenient' assessment process by the private insurance funds or a genuine reflection of the different care needs of the two groups. Given the fact that the assessment tool and protocols are standardised, perhaps it is indeed a reflection of the latter.

The eligibility criteria for each category of 'care dependency' are the same for institutional and domiciliary care and apply to those insured through public and private LTCI schemes. Commenting on the LTCI assessment process, Glendinning et al. (2004) assert that high levels of horizontal equity between older people with similar levels of care dependency are guaranteed regardless of their family or economic circumstances. High priority is given to the training of the assessors and thoroughness and uniformity of the assessment. The assessment is quite complex and is conducted by trained geriatric nurses in cooperation with a medical doctor. The assessment tool is frequently reviewed and is updated periodically to take account of new scientific and medical findings. The instrument provides information on the average amount of time it takes a person to complete certain tasks, for example, to wash, or to brush hair or teeth. While these time specifications are only meant to be used to orientate or guide nurses, criticism has been levelled at their use, since such time generalisations fail to take account of the unique circumstances of each individual.

Table 5.1 Persons acquiring domiciliary care through LTCI by category of care level and private/public insurance scheme, as of December 2003

	Public LTCI fund (%)	Private compulsory LTCI fund (%)
Care level 1	57.2	50.8
Care level 2	33.1	36.3
Care level 3	9.6	12.9

Source: Federal Ministry of Health and Social Security (2005).

A criticism frequently directed at the LTCI assessment process is that there is insufficient emphasis placed on social care. The assessment process has been criticised for focusing exclusively on physical limitations and not giving due attention to cognitive functioning (for example, persons with dementia requiring supervisory care). Awareness of this limitation has emerged at a national level and attempts have recently been made to rectify these omissions. In 2001, new legislation was introduced which provided more benefits for people with cognitive problems such as dementia. While these benefits are not very extensive at present, it appears that they will be further developed in the future. An extended assessment procedure was also introduced for persons with cognitive difficulties to take into account their special needs and requirements. As of 1 April 2002, additional funding of €460 per family per year has also become available for relatives of people with dementia. This money is to be used solely for the purpose of hiring day- or night-nurses, short-term care, general supervision services and care from recognised care providers. With limited finances and ceilings on the amount of money that can be awarded to a recipient, the extent to which further additional funding will be made is yet to be seen. Awarding 'care hours' for supervision of cognitively impaired individuals, which is currently not factored into the assessment process, would raise the costs of the LTCI programme considerably. Some critics are sceptical that such modifications in the LTCI assessment process will be made, since counting supervision hours in the assessment process would place virtually all persons with cognitive impairments in the highest-cost severe care category and costs of LTCI would thus escalate considerably (Cuellar and Wiener, 2000).

Quality Assurance

The insurance funds in association with the Medical Office of the Sickness Funds are responsible for the supervision of domiciliary care awarded through the LTCI funds. Supervision varies according to whether a recipient has had an in-kind benefit or a cash option, the latter of which is used to reward an informal family carer or other persons chosen by the care recipient such as a neighbour or friend (*Pflegegeld*). Home visits are made to beneficiaries who have chosen the cash option. The frequency of these supervision visits by a physician or nurses employed by the Medical Office is dependent on the designated care category of the LTCI recipient. For recipients in care levels 1 and 2, this check-up is done once every six months, while for those in care level 3 it occurs once every quarter, or every three months. As is the case in the assessment process, uniformity of the evaluation process is viewed as essential. The LTCI law requires that the physicians or nurses conducting the evaluation administer a universal evaluation questionnaire to all beneficiaries and that they adopt the same approach when conducting this evaluation to ensure that objectivity is guaranteed. The purpose of the visit is twofold: first, to ensure that care is adequately provided and second to explore whether the provision of certain aids or accommodation modifications could better support the care recipient and consequently reduce the number of hours of care required. The visit is also seen as an opportune time to offer an element of support and encouragement to the caregiver by promoting a dialogue between the medical specialist and the caregiver.

Supervision of the formal service providers (that is, providers who deliver care to recipients who have chosen the benefit-in-kind option) operates differently with specific legislation relating to the supervision of these providers. Since 1995, the LTCI funds have been required by the federal government to develop guidelines for assuring the quality of services provided by the service providers at the time of drawing up contracts. Further legislation in the form of the Care Quality Improvement Act, 2002, assigned responsibility for quality to the owners and managers of nursing homes and domiciliary care agencies. None the less, it would seem that adequate objective quality provisions have not been enforced and that annual negotiations between the LTCI funds and service providers more frequently focus on *price* rather than *quality* (Glendinning et al., 2004). Auditing of service providers is infrequent – by 1998 the medical office had audited only 6 per cent of all participating service providers (Cuellar and Wiener, 2000). The medical officers of the sickness funds carry out external reviews of providers when complaints are levelled against them, suggesting that in many instances the evaluation process is more reactive than proactive. Consumers'/care recipients' ability to influence the fundamental structure and subsequent quality of the LTCI scheme at the policy level is limited. Cuellar and Wiener (ibid, p. 21), commenting on this issue, argue that no accommodations are in place and that 'instead, coalitions of sickness funds negotiate with coalitions of providers without the involvement of consumers'. Figure 5.1 visually summarises the governance of the LTCI programme and the responsibilities held by different actors within the structure.

FINANCING STRUCTURE

> This is certainly one of the major challenges – how to finance the system in future. We have a pay-as-you-go system in the long-term care insurance just as in the health and pension insurance. Those working now are paying for the benefits of those who need them now. Against this backdrop, there are now demographic changes, and in the future there will be fewer people in the labour market. So who will be able to pay? And at the same time the number of recipients of these benefits will go up. This will cause us tremendous problems and we also expect a dramatic increase in dementia in the future. How we can make the system financially viable is under discussion. No political decision has been taken yet but one thing is sure, no one wants to give up long-term care insurance. (Interview with Senior Civil Servant in the Ministry of Health and Social Security, Bonn)

Unlike the United States and Denmark, provision of long-term care in Germany is not financed through income tax. Although administered by the sickness funds, long-term care is fiscally separate from acute care. LTCI is not means-tested, although social assistance to finance the costs of care over and above the benefits available via LTCI is means-tested. LTCI has one uniform contribution or premium rate of 1.7 per cent (up to an income ceiling of €3,375 per month) of gross earnings, shared equally by employers and employees. Non-employed family members are covered by the contribution of the head of household. The contributions of unemployed people are paid by their unemployment insurance. Retirees, in contrast, are obliged to pay half of the premium while the pension funds pay the other half (Cuellar and Wiener, 2000). Employers initially opposed the joint sharing of the LTCI contribution but were compensated by the elimination of one day's mandatory public holiday provided to employees. The contribution rate has not changed since the inception of the LTCI programme in 1995 and cannot be changed without an amendment to federal legislation. Annual expenditure on long-term care in 2004 amounted to approximately €8.2 billion on domiciliary care and €8.6 billion on institutional care. By law, the balance in the fund must be sufficient to enable payments to be continued for 1.5 months (Karlsson et al., 2004). Because the LTCI programme is a pay-as-you-go system, the insurance funds have not been able to build up more than a small financial balance, typically enough to cover three months (ibid.). Overall, expenditure on the programme is in line with initial expectations. Indeed, for the first few years of the programme, spending was below the estimated costs (Cuellar and Wiener, 2000).

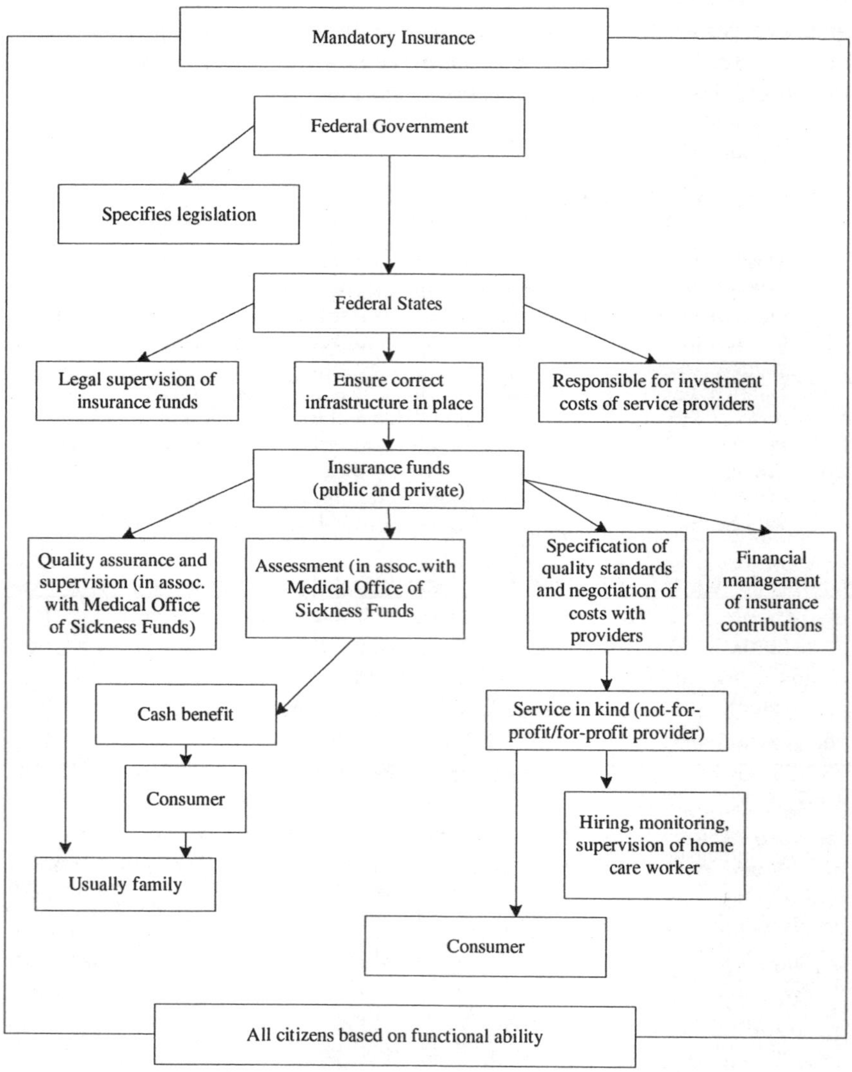

Figure 5.1 LTCI in Germany

Two factors threaten the financial sustainability of the LTCI programme as it currently functions: (i) the number of people choosing the 'cash option' may decrease and (ii) insurance premiums collected at the current contribution rate will not be sufficient to cover the future costs of the programme. As mentioned earlier, LTCI beneficiaries can choose benefits in cash or direct services provision, or a combination of both. From the outset, the viability of LTCI has been dependent on the assumption that the majority of people will choose the cash option and, indeed, to date cash has been the more popular choice. However, a higher demand for direct service provision in the context of decreased availability of family support is possible in the coming years (see below under 'Delivery Structure' for further discussion). Such an occurrence would place considerable fiscal pressure on the LTCI system. Table 5.2 indicates the maximum amount of money that an LTCI recipient can be awarded per month in each of the three care levels, and illustrates the cost savings that are made when recipients opt for the cash rather than the service option. For example, at care level 2 a cost saving of €511 per month per recipient is made when the cash option is chosen, while at care level 3 the cost saving is €767 per month per recipient. Such cost discrepancies would suggest that if an increasing number of beneficiaries choose the more costly option of direct service provision, the LTCI system would come under increasing financial pressure.

Table 5.2 Maximum payment awarded for domiciliary care according to care level and benefit option (€ per month)

	Care level 1	Care level 2	Care level 3
Benefits-in-kind	€384	€921	€1,432 (€1,918 in severe cases)
Benefits-in-cash	€205	€410	€665

Source: Federal Ministry of Health and Social Security (2005).

The second issue that may impact on the financial sustainability of the insurance programme is that the amount of money collected through the insurance premiums does not take account of inflation or that the cost (and value) of service delivery increases over time. Neither the contribution rate (1.7 per cent of gross earnings) nor the value of the payments awarded to recipients (as illustrated in Table 5.2) has changed since the programme's inception in 1995. This lack of increase in the amount awarded essentially means that the purchasing power of LTCI funds is decreasing. Based on the conservative estimate that prices for formal services increase every year by 1.5 per cent, the value of the lump sum is now 22 per cent less than it was in 1995, which in turn suggests that care recipients are not getting the same amount of services as they were getting in 1995.

Despite the fact that all insurance benefits are capped and LTCI was not conceptualised as a full-coverage insurance, it seems probable that quality of care will be compromised if neither the contribution rate nor the payment value awarded to recipients is increased in the coming years.

According to interviewees, informal discussions are under way among administrators and policy officials as to how to increase the LTCI budget. Among the solutions advanced are: (i) the creation of a citizens' insurance, which would abolish private insurance: under this proposal, everyone, including civil servants and those with high incomes, would have to contribute to the state social security system; (ii) funding through taxes rather than insurance premiums and (iii) a uniform payment rather than percentage of salary be collected from all persons.

The first suggestion that all insurance contributions be channelled into public social insurance funds only has a number of advantages. While the proportion of people who pay into the private insurance scheme is small, it is the cohort with the highest salaries and hence the highest contributions. While the benefits under LTCI through the private and public funds are equivalent, attractive private health care packages entice higher earners to the private care insurance companies. Furthermore, the premiums of the private long-term insurance funds are not related to income, but instead are related to the age of the clients when they initially sign up, thus creating an incentive for younger persons to pay into private insurance schemes (Karlsson et al., 2004). Another concern regarding the bifurcation of the insurance system is that people in the higher economic strata on average tend to be in better health than their socially disadvantaged counterparts; the latter group, who are catered for through the public funds, may require more services than the former, who are generally affiliated to the private insurance funds. This discrepancy has been borne out by the financial profits of the two sectors, with the public insurance experiencing deficits and the private a surplus. Suggestion (iii) (introduction of a uniform payment) has been advanced by the Christian Democratic party (CDU) and would ultimately only benefit higher earners who would pay lower contributions. Whatever changes are made, it is likely that employer organisations will not want the employers' mandatory contribution rate to rise, with many employer interest organisations arguing from a labour market perspective that any increases in the contribution rate should not impact on employers, who are already burdened with many non-wage labour costs that inhibit their ability to compete.

Coordinating the Costs of Long- and Short-term Care

While under the umbrella of the social insurance scheme, the LTCI programme is fiscally separate from the sickness fund,[2] which finances acute and short-term care. The sickness insurance fund still finances domiciliary care for up to four weeks where the care requirement is part of a programme of prescribed medical treatment, but only if the older person is not eligible for LTCI and no family carer is available. However, according to interviewees, at times, the boundaries between acute and long-term care can become blurred, which has resulted in problems of cost shifting and coordination between the two schemes. The separation of the LTCI scheme from the sickness insurance scheme (and consequent dichotomisation of care into short and long term) has offered few incentives to develop rehabilitation or preventive services or to improve the integration of health and social care provision (Brodsky et al., 2000; Glendinning and Igl, forthcoming). This is likely to become an issue of increasing importance in the future, given the fact that prevention (for example, falls prevention) and rehabilitation services greatly influence an individual's continuing care needs and subsequent care costs.

DELIVERY STRUCTURE

As mentioned above, cash payment as opposed to the receipt of formal service provision has been the overwhelming choice among LTCI recipients. This is, arguably, a positive indication of the willingness of families to provide care. In recent years, however, there has been a trend towards service-in-kind benefits with an increasing number of beneficiaries taking up this option, particularly as their health deteriorates. Projected increases in the number of care recipients with high levels of dependency (particularly those with cognitive impairments) coupled with expected decreases in family caregiving have caused some concern that this trend will continue, that is, an increase in the number and proportion of people who will opt for service-in-kind benefits. Additional factors such as changing household structures, geographical location,[3] economic status and relative value of cash benefits to the household budget are also likely to influence whether a beneficiary chooses the cash or service option. Between 1997 and 2001 there was a noticeable increase in the number of people choosing the service option over the cash benefit: this increase is most noticeable for LTCI beneficiaries assigned to care level 1 (least severe) (Theobald, 2005). The fact that an increasing number of lower-dependency beneficiaries are opting for the service option (or institutional care option) is an interesting development, which could suggest that either family members are not available or willing to provide care or there is a perception that delivery of formal services is preferable.

Research carried out by the German Ministry of Health, which conducted 1,001 telephone interviews with LTCI beneficiaries, provides a valuable insight into why beneficiaries may decide to choose the cash option, the service option or a combination of both (see Lundsgaard, 2005). The reasons given for choosing the cash option only included: (i) the use of the money for other miscellaneous care needs and/or (ii) not wanting to receive care from a stranger. Those who chose the service option only reported that they do so because: (i) they had no informal contacts with people who could deliver the needed care; (ii) they did not want to be a burden on their relatives; (iii) the extent of their care needs was such that they required professional assistance or (iv) a professional recommended that they take up the service option. Care recipients who chose a combination of both did so because: (i) they wanted to use the cash for miscellaneous tasks; (ii) it afforded greater flexibility and (iii) it allowed them to give a monetary payment to informal caregivers.

Cash Option: Informal (Family) Care

Germany's LTCI programme was conceived as a programme to promote and formally recognise the contribution of informal caregivers. This emphasis on and promotion of informal care is largely a consequence of its political climate, legal system and also the tradition of subsidiarity that has long been embedded in its culture and policies, especially in the area of social care. The notion of subsidiarity is a fundamental principle in the area of service provision. It means that the state should desist from performing tasks that can be fulfilled by others (most notably, the family, the church and voluntary organisations). This notion can be traced back to the Enlightenment idea that the individual has the foremost right and duty to help him/herself. In cases where this is not possible, the smallest and closest entity (that is, the family) followed by the next biggest (that is, the churches and welfare associations) should provide assistance. Only when these organisations have reached their limits, should the state intervene. This kind of thinking is still embedded in much of the relevant legislation in Germany, and in the early 1900s it was clearly visible, particularly in the areas of youth support and in social affairs, and led to a proliferation of welfare organisations (*Wohlfahrtsverbände*). The LTCI scheme also incorporates and reflects the subsidiarity principle, as it promotes the provision of care by family caregivers. Through the payment of the cash and related social security benefits, it actively incentivises informal caregiving.

More than 70 per cent of all 'care-dependent' people and 66 per cent of older 'care-dependent' people living at home rely wholly on familial care (Rothgang, 2003). In addition to the cash payment, a number of social security benefits are available to caregivers. For example, caregivers who work 14 hours or more a week, up to a maximum of 30 hours per week, earn pension credits for their work. Family caregivers are automatically covered by statutory accident insurance. If they provide at least 14 hours of care a week and have been caring for the individual for at least 12 months, they are also entitled to up to four weeks' vacation per year, during which time the sickness funds pays up to €1,432 for professional domiciliary care services. A number of social supports are also available to LTCI caregivers, such as the provision of free nursing courses for family carers. The passing of the 2002 Supplementary Law on Care Benefits (Pflegeleistungs-Ergänzungsgesetz) introduced advice and support service for carers of older people with cognitive impairments, whether LTCI beneficiaries or not.

Unfortunately, reliable statistics on which member of the social network provides care within the LTCI programme are not available. However, one indication of who these people may be was explored in the CARMA (Care for the Aged at Risk of Marginalisation) project, which analysed the provision of informal care in five countries including Germany. Overall, partners were found to constitute the largest category of family caregivers (53 per cent), but daughters or daughters-in-law were also found to offer considerable help (Table 5.3). Within the CARMA study, almost half of family caregivers reported that they were exhausted by the burden of caring. When privately hired help was utilised, it was usually for housecleaning and domestic work, or specialist care services such as physiotherapy or pedicure. Within the German sample, 40 per cent of respondents stated that these costs were covered by LTCI.

Table 5.3 Who are the informal carers in Germany?

Nature of relationship	Percentage
Daughter/Daughter-in-law	40.8
Partner (Female)	40.8
Son/Son-in-law	4.1
Partner (Male)	12.2
Other relative	2.0

Source: Abstract from Theobald (2003, p. 15).

Research has indicated that there is a visible stratification between those who choose the cash option and those who receive the services via a formal service provider based on gender, racial and socio-economic status. Studies have shown that the proportion choosing cash benefits declines with increasing disability: for instance, research by Cuellar and Wiener (2000) found that 60 per cent of the most disabled care recipients choose cash only, compared with 80 per cent of the less disabled group. After conducting a pilot study on the use of the cash allowance with the LTCI programme, Evers (1998) concluded that the allowance was used primarily to supplement the family budget and sustain informal caregiving rather than to purchase formal services. Generally, persons who are less financially secure or skilled indicate a preference for the cash option to supplement their low household budget. This viewpoint is substantiated by Dallinger (2002), who cites Mayer and Wagner's (1996) analysis of the Berlin Ageing Survey, which found that persons in higher socio-economic groups were more likely to access professional home care and, therefore, to avoid institutional care, whereas lower- and middle-class persons were more likely to access family care. Expanding on this point, Dallinger (2002, p. 6) states:

> The structure of the care insurance mainly provides incentives for women on lower incomes to act as home-carers. For women with higher income and professional status the low cash benefits are not a real incentive to care at home. In contrast, it is a strong incentive for non-employed women that they are integrated into the social insurance system if they provide care for an elderly relative. For them as well as for women in unattractive, low paid jobs, the cash for care work is an option.

At a national level the government has formally recognised the importance of supporting informal caregivers and an active self-help community organisation landscape. However, while the law empowers the *Länder* to offer community-run activity programmes which support caregivers, they are not obliged to do so. Since these programmes are generally run on a voluntary basis, there are large regional variations in their availability, with better service infrastructure usually available in more economically advantaged areas. If the continued dependence on informal caregivers within the LCTI programme continues, it would seem that the further promotion and availability of community service support schemes is essential to the further success and sustainability of the programme.

Formal Service Providers

> If you look at social welfare or at youth services or youth programmes the law specifies that the state should cooperate with social welfare organisations. And this is a privilege which was eliminated in the law on long-term care insurance and was done with some emphasis. This means that those offering the service under the long-term care insurance are not only the welfare organisations but also the umbrella organisations of private suppliers. (Interview at the Senate for Health, Social Affairs and Consumer Protection)

Historically, providers sponsored by charitable welfare organisations received special treatment by the *Länder* and were the dominant suppliers of long-term care services. The principle of subsidiarity (referred to above) asserts that once a family's caregiving capabilities have been exhausted the next most acceptable provider is the church or welfare organisation. The notion of subsidiarity was enshrined in the Federal Social Assistance Act of 1961, which privileged Germany's six welfare associations[4] in the delivery of social services and obliged local authorities to offer support and assistance to these organisations: local authorities were forbidden to supply social services that could be delivered by welfare organisations. The LTCI legislation, however, ended the privileged position of the welfare organisations in the delivery of long-term care and required insurance funds to treat both the not-for-profit and for-profit organisations equally and to favour them over public agencies. This has meant that the welfare organisations no longer enjoy market monopoly as they had done previously. Bönker and Wollmann (2005, p. 15), commenting on the new model of service delivery, state:

> [T]raditional local government has been seized by a rampant flux towards 'corporatisation', 'outsourcing' and 'privatisation' . . . the close and exclusive co-operation with the welfare associations has been replaced with more transparent behaviour and a more market-like management of contracts with a plethora of different providers.

Service-in-kind beneficiaries can choose between any of the provider organisations that have contracts with their LTCI fund. Any provider who fulfils certain prerequisites is entitled to get a service contract with the insurance funds. However, in 2002, it was ruled that only providers who introduce internal quality management practices would get a contract with the insurance funds. There are over 11,000 private and not-for-profit domiciliary care providers, with only 4 per cent of care delivered through the LTCI system being delivered by public sector care providers (Schneekloth and Müller, 2000). The proliferation of the private home care sector is apparent from figures presented by Bönker and Wollmann (2005), who estimate that the number of professional domiciliary care providers more than doubled from approximately 6,000 in 1995 to 12,695 in 2003, and that the number of employees in domiciliary and institutional care increased from 270,000 in 1996 to 665,000 in 2001. Currently, more than half of the service providers are private: however, it is estimated that 63 per cent of the care contracted out via the LTCI programme is to the not-for-profit sector (Theobald, 2005). The reason for this is that private organisations tend to be small,[5] while the welfare associations continue to be very large. In other words, while there are more private domiciliary care providers, the welfare associations have the most employees and clients and thus still control the larger proportion of the market (see Table 5.4). Currently, there does not seem to be a proportionate supply of service provider: in some urban areas there is more supply than demand, while the converse is true in more rural areas. Private organisations tend to be more plentiful in urban densely populated areas. For example, in Hamburg, Berlin and Bremen, between 61.9 and 74.9 per cent of all providers are classified as private (ibid.).

Table 5.4 Providers of formal care in Germany

	Private for-profit	Private not-for-profit	Public
Number	5,594	5,103	213
Percentage share of all providers	51	47	2
Average number of dependent persons cared for	27	51	37

Source: Brodsky et al. (2000, p. 34) citing StBA (2001, p. 11).

The for-profit and not-for-profit providers compete in a highly regulated market. This competition is not 'free' in the sense of the operation of normal free markets because there are many predefined criteria and conditions which the providers have to fulfil, and the LTCI funds have to provide comparative price lists to LTCI beneficiaries. Providers do not have an opportunity to set their own prices; rather they must discuss this with the insurance funds and negotiate a price that the fund is willing to pay. According to interviewees one intention behind this price negotiating was that prices would be controlled for persons who require additional care over that which had been awarded via the LTCI programme – controlling the prices in this way may enable more people to purchase supplementary formal care services. Every provider is free to engage in negotiations directly with the care insurance fund. If agreements cannot be reached, a special arbitration board consisting of members from both sides is convened to agree on a price (Rothgang, 2003). According to Rothgang, these discussions tend to revolve more around the number of credit points a particular task involves than the outcome of care. For every task, there are a certain number of credit points. The value of the credit point is the result of negotiations between the social insurance fund and the service provider and the value depends on the specific task required, for example, one provider may offer a marginally cheaper service to bathe than to dress a client and vice versa.

According to interviewees the insurance funds are open to negotiation when estimating these costs, and providers can request higher payment for a service if they can prove that they can offer a better quality service. However, the scope for negotiation is limited as the amount agreed cannot exceed the standard rate by a wide margin and, as a result, the increases agreed are usually minimal, for example, 3.1 cents instead of 3 cents. New elements of competition between the not-for-profit and for-profit agencies have caused some tension that usually relates to cost of service and one provider's insistence that their overhead costs are greater than another's. Some organisations argue that their higher costs result from better-trained, higher-quality staff, while a number of private operators argue that they have higher overhead costs (including start-up costs) than the welfare organisations,[6] which they argue the federal government should cover. In 2005, the umbrella group of private providers (Bundesverband Privater Anbieter sozialer Dienste) joined with the umbrella group of the welfare organisations (Bundesarbeitsgemeinschaft der Freien Wohlfahrtspflege, and Deutscher Pflegerat) to document their grievances, which included: (i) that the definition of care is too narrow and (ii) that the amount of money available at each care level is too low and needs to rise in accordance with inflation levels. They also called for a reduction in bureaucracy and regulation of investment costs at national level. At the federal level, the private providers also demanded increased funding towards start-up costs.

Care Workforce Issues

The LTCI law states that senior personnel within home care provider organisations must have appropriate qualifications, usually nursing qualifications. Paramedical care such as injections and treatment of wounds can only be conducted by such qualified persons. While there are no minimum training qualifications for domiciliary care workers, the law states that their work must be supervised by a qualified nurse. The introduction of the LTCI programme coincided with an increase in employment rates for qualified staff. However, as Theobald (2003, p. 167) notes, less-skilled care workers are 'over-represented within marginal, part-time employment, which very often leaves them without any type of basic social security cover'. This stratification of the workforce is becoming increasingly evident in both the for-profit and welfare organisations, where more senior or qualified staff receive a higher remuneration at the expense of the lower-skilled workers. Payment scales are recommended within the German labour market tariff system, although these scales are not mandatory and generally are not used by the private providers.

Interviews conducted in the course of this project suggest that some welfare organisations are also no longer complying with public service salaries and benefits. However, the impact of these cuts is generally most pronounced for less-skilled employees.

CONSUMER POWER

Domiciliary care recipients within the LTCI system have been granted consumer *choice* but little consumer *direction*. Care recipients are given a choice of cash benefits (to be paid to an informal caregiver) or service provision from a formal service provider. With regard to the latter, they can also choose whether the service provider will be a private provider or a not-for-profit or welfare organisation. Furthermore, care recipients who opt for the cash benefits are given the choice of employing a friend, relative or neighbour. The OECD (2005, p. 55), commenting on the level of consumer control in the German long-term care system, points out:

> While there are no explicit restrictions on how the German Cash Allowance for Care is spent, the older person and their relatives are nevertheless obliged to acquire sufficient care . . . if older people are found to be receiving insufficient care in light of their needs, the authorities must make some in-kind provision of care services, in which case the cash allowance will be withdrawn.

Recipients who opt for the in-kind option can receive only services from the providers who have contracts with the insurance funds and are generally awarded care by care task rather than for a specified period. This means that consumer *direction* is virtually absent: recipients are awarded a specific care task and, unlike care recipients in Denmark, cannot suggest an alternative task, that is, the ability to change or direct the work of the care worker is limited. In Germany, a certain predefined care package is awarded. Prior to the introduction of the LTCI programme, care delivered through the social security system was very often awarded in units of time. The system, as it currently functions, is less flexible with the care worker calling at the care recipient's house to complete a specified task, irrespective of whether this is the most essential requirement of the client on that particular day.

According to interviewees in the Ministry of Health a number of pilot projects are currently under way to explore whether consumer direction can be extended with the expansion of the cash benefit option and the introduction of a cash-for-care model. While administrators and policy officials can see many advantages of a system that enables care recipients to define their own care needs, there is also an awareness that such a system would necessitate professional advice and monitoring by case managers to ensure that funds are spent sensibly and that quality services are delivered. It is expected that results of these pilot projects will be available in 2008.

CONCLUSIONS

Germany has a long tradition of social insurance. Prior to 1994, however, there was no comprehensive system of funding long-term care: access to many services was means-tested and local governments had the responsibility for financing these. The LTCI legislation of 1994 granted universal rights to long-term care funding for all persons who satisfy specified functional criteria. The reform was successful in removing considerable fiscal pressure from the local governments and in providing a basic level of assistance to persons in need of long-term care. In short, the introduction of LTCI constituted a fundamental shift from a system based on the local social assistance schemes to a national and universal insurance programme.

As a result of the introduction of LTCI, local governments no longer exercise the same level of control over the provision of long-term care services in their community. The introduction of the LTCI scheme has passed on the responsibility for the eligibility process, the contracting process and quality control to the care insurance funds. The traditional ties that bound local government with welfare organisations have been loosened with the introduction of the LTCI scheme, resulting in a changing landscape of service provision, with the virtual monopoly of welfare organisations being replaced by a more level playing field and the proportion of private service providers to welfare organisations almost balancing out in certain areas.

The LTCI programme is faced with a number of challenges. It is heavily reliant on the continued contributions of informal caregivers and the fact that the majority of recipients opt for the 'cheaper' (to the public purse) cash option. With a rise in care recipients with higher levels of dependency, a decline in familial caregiving, and no change in either the insurance contribution payments or the value of the cash payment, the LTCI scheme, as it currently operates, is likely to run into fiscal problems in the coming years unless modifications are made. A further difficulty is the fact that the LTCI funds currently operate on capped budgets and do not cover the full cost of care. For this reason, a large proportion of LTCI beneficiaries have to pay out-of-pocket costs to supplement care received through the LTCI programme. Another challenge that has emerged since the introduction of the LTCI programme is the fact that responsibility for long-term care and acute care was separated. As a consequence, there has been little incentive to better integrate and coordinate rehabilitative services (coordinated through the sickness insurance funds) with long-term care services. Despite these limitations, there seems to be widespread consensus that the LTCI programme has been a success, the coverage of care needs has been expanded, strict implementation of national standards has introduced an element of horizontal equity hitherto not possible and the contribution of informal caregivers has been recognised, consequently providing them with pay, respite, social security benefits and better support. As a result, Germany's LTCI system may serve as a useful example for other countries considering the creation of a national LTCI programme.

NOTES

1. See www.bmgs.bund.de/eng/gra/4294.php.
2. The sickness funds are quasi-public, quasi-private insurers that are regulated at a national level: while contributions are mandatory, premiums vary between individual insurers (unlike in the

case of LTCI) (Cuellar and Wiener, 2000).

3. Research by Dallinger (2002) found that there was a higher use of formal care services in the former East Germany compared with the West: while 43 per cent of LTCI recipients accessed formal services in the East, this was the case for only 30 per cent in the West.

4. Innere Mission/Diakonie (Lutheran); Deutscher Caritas-Verband (Catholic); Arbeiterwohlfahrt (Social-Democratic/workers); Deutsches Rotes Kreuz (German Red Cross); Paritätischer Wohlfahrtsverband (Independent); and Zentralwohlfahrverband der deuschen Juden (Jewish).

5. Schneeklooth and Müller (2000) note that 17 per cent of private organisations have fewer than five employees.

6. The welfare organisations are financed through a mix of sources such as user fees, membership contributions, public subsidies, private donations and investment incomes (Aust et al., 2002).

6. Delivery of Home Care: Observation of Services on the Ground

> Domiciliary care takes place in a special space, that of home. We need to grasp the meaning of this and by consequence, the significance of care workers coming into that space. Home is also structured in terms of time, and the patterns of this can clash with the logic of service provision, based as it is on a different form of time and a different, service-based, rationality. (Twigg, 2000, p. viii)

Most of the comparative literature on domiciliary care services focuses on the issue at a macro level, examining the financing, delivery structure and legal framework in which it is posited. Little or no effort has been made to elucidate the reality of domiciliary care services from the perspective of the older person, that is, the home care recipient, or from the perspective of the home care workers. Due to budgetary and time constraints, it was not possible to conduct an in-depth, comparative analysis of the domiciliary care services from the perspective of care recipients and care workers within this study. However, three observation exercises were arranged in each of the three countries to gain a cursory insight into the day-to-day reality of the respective domiciliary care systems.

Observational methods were chosen for this study because of the short time-frame available to the researchers in each of the three research sites, and because of language difficulties that might be encountered. The scheduling of the observation exercises was arranged prior to the fieldwork trips with key administrative players in each of the respective countries.

In Denmark and Germany, the care recipients were not, in most cases, completely aware that the observer was a social science researcher. In Denmark the home care worker introduced the researcher to care recipients and in Germany the researcher introduced herself to care recipients. However, the brevity of each visit did not permit an in-depth introduction. As a consequence, many care recipients viewed the researcher as a trainee home care worker or a nurse. In retrospect, this was somewhat advantageous, as it meant that the majority of home care recipients did not feel that they, or the interaction between them and the home care worker, were being observed. After each observation exercise the researcher wrote a narrative record detailing each visit or meeting. This included notes relating to the age and health status of care recipients and the home environment. Where possible, conversations and interactions between care workers and home care recipients were also recorded. Where the researcher believed her presence might be somewhat intrusive, such as when personal care needs were being attended to, agreement was sought from both the care recipient and the care worker as to the appropriateness of her presence.

The observation data are presented below in two parts. First, a brief synopsis of a small number of the visits in Denmark, the United States and Germany is presented. This section provides a cursory insight into the domiciliary care world in the three settings and elucidates the different contexts within which each of the home care workers operate. Second, a comparative analysis of the three settings is provided. This section takes a more comparative focus. It examines the duties of the home care worker, the work environment and the levels of monitoring and support received by the care worker and the issue of informal care. These case studies are not completely comparable but they do offer a window into the uncharted world of domiciliary care services at the front-line.[1]

OBSERVATION OF DOMICILIARY CARE WORK

Denmark

Home care worker: pseudonym, Helena

This observation exercise was arranged with a public domiciliary care worker through the assistance of the Danish Trade Union of Public Employees (Forbundet af Offentligt Ansatte or FOA).

The day began at 7.30 a.m. in the staffroom of a public sector home care organisation in a Copenhagen suburb. There were 15 home care workers seated around a table drinking their morning coffee. Each care worker was given a handout with a list of clients for the day. The number of minutes per client and type of care required were also outlined on these handouts. Five-minute intervals were allocated between each client and an additional 45 minutes was allocated to each worker to allow for any unexpected delays during the day. A brief three- to four-minute exchange took place between some of the care workers about their workload for the day.

Helena had nine calls to make: all of her clients were within close proximity of each other and none was more than eight minutes cycling distance away. She had a key for each of the clients and at the entrance to the building she first rang the bell and then made her way to the apartment. Each visit lasted between 20 and 30 minutes. Helena's care duties differed according to the needs of the clients; rather than go through each of the nine visits in detail, three visits of varying types are summarised below.

Visit 1 On leaving one care recipient, we went to the care recipient's next-door neighbours, an elderly married couple in their nineties. The man had great difficulty walking, only doing so with the aid of crutches. When we entered the apartment, the couple were sitting side-by-side looking out of the window. The woman explained that her husband had had a mishap the night before, due to incontinence, and asked Helena if she could check on him and tend to his care needs. Before Helena did this, she went with the woman to fix her hair. The woman sat by the mirror and Helena took down her hair, brushed it and put it in a neat bun. Helena then quickly made the bed and asked the man to join her in the kitchen. The apartment was small and there was not enough room in the bathroom for her to wash the man, so she carried out this task in the kitchen where, propped on a little stool, Helena washed the man as he stood leaning against the sideboard. He then sat down and she fastened his clothes. His wife closely supervised Helena as she completed personal care tasks. Later, Helena told me that the man has found it very difficult to come to terms with his disability and has become very antisocial and frustrated by his weekly visit to the day centre. Helena believed that if the wife were not alive he would not be able to remain living at home as his care needs are too great.

Visit 2 We then cycled to a social housing complex, which was approximately a seven-minute cycle ride from our previous visit. Our appointment was with a woman belonging to an ethnic minority community, who was partly paralysed; she had no English or Danish and seemed to be experiencing quite a bit of pain. We entered the woman's room, which resembled a hospital room rather than a bedroom. The woman, who was extremely frail, weighing no more than five stones, was lying in a hospital-style bed. A nurse who had just administered an insulin injection was leaving as we entered the apartment. Another home help (male) was also present as two care workers were always necessary whenever visits were made to this woman, due to the fact that she was immobile and lifting was usually required. The two domiciliary care workers washed the woman as she lay in bed: this demanded considerable effort, she seemed to be in pain whenever she was moved. Rolling her gently onto each side, they bathed her and changed her incontinence pad. They then washed her upper body and face. Throughout the bathing exercise, the woman moaned, all the time speaking in her native tongue. Her eyes were very alert, constantly moving and staring with a look of apparent fear at the person standing beside her. Once bathing was complete, Helena crushed some tablets, which the woman took without objection.

Helena explained later that this woman did not like the domiciliary care workers or nurses visiting her. The woman is exceptional in that she has very high care needs and still lives at home. The reason for this is that the family do not want her to go into a nursing home, believing that this would reflect badly on them. The domiciliary care workers deliver only personal care to this woman while the family are responsible for other care duties, including domestic help and food preparation. The woman receives a visit from a domiciliary care worker six times a day, in addition to daily visits from a nurse.

We visited this woman again after lunch (once again accompanied by another home care worker). The woman's daughter-in-law had just fed her. This time the visit was very short – the woman's incontinence pad was checked and since it was still dry no additional care was needed.

Visit 3 We then made our way to an assisted living complex. We met with a woman who looked very fresh and agile. The tasks in this house were to wash the dishes, make the bed and help put on the woman's supportive stockings. The visit, which lasted 15 to 20 minutes, was very cordial and the home care worker and the woman chatted together in a friendly manner. In some respects, the visit also seemed to serve as a 'check-up and greeting' visit.

Other visits Additional calls made during the day were to a woman with obsessive-compulsive disorder and arthritis in her hand. Under careful supervision, Helena washed and prepared carrots, parsnips, broccoli and garlic for the woman to cook later on. Light domestic chores (making the bed and washing dishes) were done for a man also living in an assisted living dwelling. Lunch was prepared for another woman in her seventies, while the purpose of another visit was the administration/supervision of medication. An afternoon return visit to the woman with obsessive-compulsive disorder was cancelled as the woman had made an appointment to see an eye specialist and did not require Helena's assistance.

At lunchtime we returned to the centre where once again all of the domiciliary care workers had gathered round a table. After lunch, the manager asked the care workers about their morning, and the care workers exchanged stories about their morning shift as well as about the health status of various clients. Helena spoke about the woman with obsessive-compulsive disorder and the woman from an ethnic minority community, the most demanding visits of the morning. After the staff meeting, which lasted about 15 minutes, the domiciliary care workers went back to do the final two calls of the day. Helena told me that she enjoys the light-duty visits that involve just washing the dishes and making the bed as they give her time to relax and daydream before seeing a more labour-intensive client. Helena's workday finished at 2.30 p.m. Before finishing, she returned the worksheet she had received that morning which she had updated during the day. This worksheet recorded the amount of time she had spent with each client and any pertinent issues that arose during the visit.

Of the eight visits made in Denmark, more than half of the clients lived in assisted living dwellings. These varied from an old-style two-roomed apartment to a brightly lit, modern and spacious four-roomed apartment looking out on to an open green area. The advantages of this assisted living accommodation were apparent. From the perspective of the care worker, work was contained within a small area. From the point of view of the care recipients, there was a resident warden on call in case of any concerns.

San Francisco

Home care recipient: pseudonym, Stacy; home care worker: pseudonym, Cleo

This exercise was scheduled via the PA. Instead of an observation exercise, interviews were completed to facilitate the wishes of both the IHSS care worker and care recipient. The section below details these meetings, first from the perspective of the IHSS recipient, and then from the perspective of the IHSS care worker.

Stacy's story (IHSS home care recipient) Stacy became disabled in 1990 and was assigned a social worker who informed her about the IHSS. As she did not know of anyone who would work for her she was assigned a care worker through the IHSS contract or agency mode. Initially, the care worker came to her house for three hours every day but did not visit at weekends. At this time she lived with her mother who took care of her and her father who also had a disability. The fact that her father had a disability had no bearing on Stacy getting a care worker to call at the weekends. As soon as the PA was established, Stacy switched to the independent provider (IP) contract mode. Once she switched over to the IP mode, she was awarded more hours from the Department of Human Services and was able to hire someone for the mornings and weekends. Stacy currently has three home care workers; one has worked for her for eight years, another for two years and another for just four months. One care worker visits in the mornings, another visits in the evening and the third comes to her home at weekends. In total, she receives 171.3 hours of care per month.

When approached, the PA provided Stacy with a list of potential care workers. Stacy prioritised them according to whether they smoked as well as their proximity as she wanted a care worker who lived in the vicinity. Sometimes, it was necessary to go through two or three lists before a suitable worker could be found. There are a number of attributes that Stacy believes to be essential for a home care worker. Most of all, she believes that patience, an altruistic nature and empathy are crucial characteristics: 'They have to have some empathy, 'cause if they don't have that, they really can't learn the job'.

Stacy has had some bad experiences with home care workers but dislikes having to fire a worker. When a worker is fired, it is difficult to find someone else. She finds the IHSS manual, which offers advice on hiring and firing, useful in this regard. A social worker visits once a year to see whether anything needs to be changed and whether Stacy needs more hours. In the event of her health deteriorating and Stacy needing more help, she will contact her physician and ask him to outline her difficulties. However, her experiences with physicians have largely been negative, and she believes that if she is not direct with them, instructing them what to write, the physician: 'will write some gobbledy-gook that you have to have someone else interpret for you and they would end up sending the letter back to me saying they need another explanation'.

The social workers issue a letter specifying the number of hours awarded with a list of the recommended chores that should be done (for example, eight hours a month for meal preparation). Stacy usually abides by the amount of time they have outlined for each task, but explained that the ability to stick to this time-frame is influenced by the home care workers, with some being more efficient than others. Stacy prefers to be structured and organised and likes to inform her care workers in advance of the jobs they will do during the week. She explained that home care recipients have to be very organised:

> You have so many different people in your house you have to have everything where you know it is going to be. So when I ask a worker to look for a spatula I always keep the spatula in the same drawer so I know where everything is.

The care workers who come in the mornings and weekends do most of the chores and most of the personal care work. The evening care worker does light housework, prepares the meals and provides some personal care. Stacy has over 50 cookbooks; she is very interested in cooking and likes to cook 'vicariously' through her care workers.

In the event of a care worker being sick, Stacy has to use the PA's on-call service. She does not think that this service is very efficient and expressed concern that most of the people on the registry are immigrants who are not proficient English speakers. Despite the fact that she speaks slowly and distinctly to them, she believes that: 'they only hear what they want to hear, so language is a problem'. Also, she is wary about letting strangers into her house, saying she does not operate a revolving-door policy, and generally likes to have met the care worker before they start working for her.

Stacy prefers the IP mode to the contract mode:

> I rather pick and choose who I would like to come into my home. I think I would have to be at a point where I couldn't judge for myself, then I would opt for the Consortium mode and then if it went beyond that I would have to have a conservator. But I think the IP mode lets me be independent and do as much as I can.

She did, however, acknowledge that the IP mode does not suit everyone, listing frail older people and persons with dementia as two groups that may not be suited to the responsibility expected in the IP mode. She stated that there is nothing she would change about the IHSS IP mode. However, she believes that higher wages and stable benefits for the care workers are essential as this would help to entice and retain a higher calibre care worker. Additionally, she is not an advocate of mandatory training and likes to be able to train her workers herself: ''cause those who already know what to do are harder to work with'.

Cleo's story (IHSS home care worker) When Cleo's mother became ill a number of years ago, Cleo started helping her at home, whenever possible. When her mother was admitted to hospital, a social worker talked to her about who would take care of her mother on her return home. Cleo, surprised by the question, informed the social worker that she would and was then told that she could get paid through the IHSS programme for doing so. Once her mother recovered, Cleo wanted to help somebody else, so she contacted the PA and asked for her name to be included on its registry. Shortly thereafter, Stacy received Cleo's contact information and hired her. Cleo now has three clients: 'each with different needs but basically all the same, just basic domestic stuff, like clean up and stuff that they can't do'. Among the duties she does for Stacy are cooking, helping her get dressed, toileting and helping her with grooming. When her mother was sick she explained she had to do: 'the same stuff you do in a hospital. We just don't get paid like they get paid'. Cleo explained that she enjoys taking care of people, especially when working for clients such as Stacy, her mother and Ms Drury (an older woman whom she cares for).

When she first started working for Stacy, Cleo worked only at weekends, for a total of 36 hours a month. Now she works Monday to Friday and the hours have doubled. She worked 82 hours a month for her mother and over 80 hours for Ms Drury. She explained that sometimes she has worked with care recipients who were awarded only a small number of hours per month. However, it is this flexibility that attracts her to the job, as she finds work does 'not consume all my time'.

Cleo has a good working relationship with her clients, so if she ever needs to reschedule the time of a visit, her clients are generally flexible. Conversely, if her clients request additional hours at short notice, she is usually happy to accommodate them. This cooperative relationship, as well as improving work relationships and job satisfaction, can also bring benefits at important festive times:

> 'cause it's more than I'm her client and she's my provider and vice versa, it's more than that with my clients. Like I have a client in the hospital now and I go see her everyday 'cause you know it's more than just working for them. And that goes back to you have to like what you do. And she don't even like me to

> work on holidays 'cause I have children so it works out well once you like who you're working for and who's working for you likes you.

Cleo believes that patience is essential when working as a home care worker. She pointed out that Stacy likes duties to be done slowly to ensure that everything is done correctly, so she cannot rush her chores. She believes that the job is more like a vocation, and a desire to care for people is essential if you are to stay in the job. She has little to no contact with the PA, as: 'all my directions come from my clients, 'cause they are my boss'. Cleo enjoys cooking for Stacy and has learned new culinary skills. She relayed how she now enjoys cooking for her own family and likes to show off new recipes that she has learned from Stacy.

Cleo is aware that the conditions for IHSS workers have improved dramatically in the past few years. She has health and dental insurance but laments the fact that her children are covered on this policy only for dental expenses and not for medical expenses. In her last job her children were covered for medical expenses, something that she thinks is more important that dental insurance. If she wanted to she could work full-time, but she is aware that there is a limit on the total number of hours the Department of Health will allow a care worker to do. She covers transport costs herself.

Cleo believes that the IHSS is an invaluable service and that the suitability of the IP mode is related to the severity of disability. She expressed concern that the maximum number of hours allocated is sometimes not adequate and, consequently, families have to pay out of pocket to get additional care. She relayed how a friend of her mother's had Alzheimer's disease and needed round-the-clock care. The friend's son, unable to provide 24-hour care, hired additional family members to supervise his mother. Although this was an informal arrangement, his relatives insisted that they get paid the same salary as an IHSS worker.

Germany

Observation exercises proved somewhat difficult to arrange in Germany. More than ten individual welfare organisations were contacted and after considerable effort an observation exercise was arranged with a fluent English speaker in one large welfare organisation. The first observation involved accompanying a domiciliary care nurse. A brief observation exercise with a domiciliary care worker proficient in English (employed in the same organisation) also took place. The first summary below details the observation exercise conducted with the home care nurse, the second with the home care worker.

Home care nurse: pseudonym, Hilda

A meeting was arranged for 6.45 a.m. at the domiciliary care centre on the outskirts of Berlin. While Hilda's shift begins at 7.00 a.m., she explained that she comes in at 6.40 a.m. each morning to do paperwork and organise the different medications that she will distribute during the course of the day. She explained that some of the care workers begin work at 5.40 a.m. Hilda always goes by car as she has a considerable distance to cover. She explained that there is a lot of pressure on her to be punctual. Every day she registers the time and duration of her visits and outlines the reasons for any delays. As a nurse, she is paid a fixed monthly salary, unlike domiciliary care workers who are paid weekly based on the number of calls they make. She believed that some of the care recipients she visited also had domiciliary care workers calling, but she was unsure of which care recipients these were.

In total we visited 14 clients, all of whom seemed to have very different needs. Unlike the Danish observation exercise, these visits were shorter in duration, lasting between 10 and 20 minutes; four of these visits are outlined below.

Visit 1 We put on plastic boots before entering the house of a woman in her eighties from an ethnic minority community. She lived in a relatively new social housing complex, in a very bare, but clean apartment. The woman had neither German nor English, however, Hilda said that she is able to tell whether the woman was in pain or not. In addition to receiving care via long-term care insurance (LTCI), the woman also received social welfare assistance. According to Hilda, the woman's son is supposed to be looking after her and receives LTCI benefits, however, in Hilda's opinion, the care the son gives to his mother is inadequate. The woman suffers from severe constipation. She believed that the woman's symptoms would not be so severe if her son fed her less processed and more fibrous foods. During the visit the woman was trying to relay something in her native language. Hilda did not understand, so she phoned the son who spoke English. He explained that he was taking his mother to the doctor that day. Hilda helped the woman wash herself and made the bed; she explained that making the bed is not something she would usually do, but she knew that the son would not do it. Before leaving, she checked the woman's medicine cabinet and noticed that she was low on certain medication; she ordered this medication over the phone, which she would subsequently deliver to the woman.

Visit 2 The next visit was to a woman in her late seventies who was recently diagnosed with diabetes. On entering the house, Hilda greeted her with a kiss on the cheek, something she did with almost all of her clients, and which she believed was very unusual for a home nurse or domiciliary care worker. She explained that she feels very attached to all her clients and likes to greet them in such a manner on each visit. For the past few weeks Hilda has been visiting this woman to teach her how to self-inject. The woman was going on holiday for two weeks and needed to know how to administer her own insulin injections. The meeting lasted approximately ten minutes and was informal and chatty.

Visit 3 This visit was to a man who had been discharged from hospital and had just been awarded care through the LTCI programme. The man's feet were noticeably dirty and considerably infected. He explained that he had been living in his present home for 20 years and that he disliked his experience in hospital and was glad to be back in familiar surroundings. Hilda later commented that the hospital had not adequately cleaned the man's infected feet. This was Hilda's first meeting with the man, so she introduced herself and asked him a few brief questions, while she cleaned his feet. She explained that it would take four to five weeks before they would heal properly. Hilda queried whether he had any family to help him. He said that he had two daughters who visited once a week with shopping. However, Hilda was sceptical of this and believed that the man was very much neglected. Because it was the first visit there was an extensive list of questions that Hilda had to ask and complete on a form, which would subsequently be sent to the LTCI funding organisation.

Visit 4 Following that visit, we called on a woman in her late eighties who had dementia, diabetes and a hearing problem. Tragically, her son who was her carer had been diagnosed with cancer and was in hospital. The woman's niece was taking the place of the son while he was in hospital. The woman required daily insulin injections, but the niece was unable to administer these and so had called upon the nurse to do so. The niece was very anxious about her aunt, and seemed upset and stressed, and looked noticeably tired. The accommodation was very small and cramped, and there was an aura of tension and claustrophobia in the apartment. The woman sat in her living-room chair, apparently lost in her own incomprehensible utterances, while Hilda administered the insulin injection and chatted with the woman's niece, who informed Hilda that she was gravely concerned about her aunt. The visit lasted only five to six minutes.

Other comments For each of the clients she visited, Hilda had to fill out a form – she explained that these forms are sent to the insurance companies and are tedious and time-consuming. Hilda generally has the same clients who are rotated between her and another nurse. She commented that at times her colleague was not able to keep up with her workload and Hilda often has to make additional calls to these clients. As we drove between clients, Hilda explained that she enjoys her job, because she likes caring for people and making them happy. Occasionally, however, she sees family members whom she believes abuse the system and felt that it is easier for families to renege on caregiving duties than it is for a professional care worker, and that some families want to take the money but do not want to pay for services.

On our journey between visits, we passed two vans that supply hot meals to older people. These operations are run by private companies and charge up to €6.00 or €7.00 per meal. Hilda explained that this is very expensive for the majority of older people, so often these meals are purchased as a treat. However, she said that for others, who are unable to cook, it is a necessity.

Home care worker: pseudonym, Marie

Marie is in her mid-sixties and cycles to all her clients since she does not own a car. She has been working for the home care organisation since 1995; before that she worked as a domestic help for ten years in the home of an English commandant living in Berlin. She said she enjoys her work, as the care recipients become her friends. The only time she does not like the job is when colleagues are sick or are unable to visit all their clients, which means that she has a heavier caseload. She works five days a week, sometimes weekends, but then she will have two days off during the week to compensate for the weekend work. Weekend work is usually easier, as care workers are not allowed to bathe care recipients or shop for food; work at weekends usually entails getting the person out of bed and preparing a light meal. Generally, Marie starts at 7 a.m. and has roughly one hour per care recipient. She has been visiting some of the care recipients for a long time, but they are also frequently rotated. That morning she had been to visit two clients: the first visit involved helping the client out of bed, prompting medication, helping with bathing and changing the incontinence pad; the second involved helping the client out of bed and preparing breakfast.

Visit 1 This visit was to the house of a 72-year-old client who lived in a two-roomed apartment. The apartment was small but cosy, with a heavy stench of cigarette smoke. There was a pet guinea pig in a cage in the corner, which seemed to give the woman a tremendous amount of pleasure. Marie and the home care recipient drew up a shopping list of goods that Marie would purchase. The woman then gave Marie €50 shopping money. The domiciliary care worker usually cycles to the shop, which takes approximately five minutes, however, walking as we did took 15 minutes. On the way to the shop we bumped into another domiciliary care worker, who shares a roster with Marie. They spoke about a number of their clients, including one who did not have enough money to do the shopping because the son had spent it. We then spent ten minutes in the shop and also brought plastic bottles to the recycling bank.

When we returned to the woman's house, Marie explained that her brief was to vacuum the apartment, but the woman, who was a very jovial person, said there was no need and invited Marie to sit down instead. The domiciliary care worker seemed to agree that the apartment was adequately clean, but none the less, decided that it should be vacuumed. Even though Marie and the woman had known each other for only one month, their relationship was very informal and friendly and they seemed to genuinely enjoy each other's company.

Visit 2 The next client lived approximately a ten-minute drive away. This client, who had advanced cancer, was sitting watching television in her underwear and T-shirt when we entered. Marie had already visited her early that morning and had changed her incontinence pad and prompted her to take her medication. The purpose of this visit was once again to change her pad and to prepare some food. However, the woman said she did not need her pad changed and also said that she would be able to make her own lunch. Marie explained that up to one week ago, the woman was completely immobile, but in the last week has managed to walk with the help of a walking aid. We did the washing up from breakfast. Marie also had to clean the bathroom and mop the kitchen floor. When she went to flush the toilet, the pipe in the toilet burst and overflowed, and, consequently, we spent the best part of 15 minutes mopping up the water. Once this was done and the kitchen floor cleaned, Marie had finished her chores. Conversation between Marie and the client was minimal. Whether this was normal or a consequence of the observation exercise was difficult to ascertain. Marie then went into the bedroom where the client's files were stored and completed the record sheets, outlining what she had done during the visit, and explaining that the toilet had overflowed.

COMPARATIVE ANALYSIS OF THE THREE OBSERVATION EXERCISES

Home Care Workers' Duties

The job of a home care worker, as can be gleaned from the observation exercises described above, is a very versatile one. Tasks were broad-ranging with care workers generally working in a dual capacity, doing light domestic work and providing personal care. Domestic work included help with food preparation, cleaning and shopping. Personal care generally related to helping people out of bed, help with dressing, prompting medication, bathing, application of ointments, showering and grooming. In addition, care workers provided companionate care ranging from conversational and emotional support to respite and supervisory care for persons with dementia (see Figure 6.1 for summary of different tasks).

Medical conditions of the home care recipients ranged from psychiatric illness, dementia and anxiety to strokes, diabetes, cancer, multiple sclerosis, paralysis and respiratory and mobility problems. The Danish home care worker provided help with domestic tasks, including food preparation, cleaning the bedroom and kitchen, as well as personal care in the form of supervision of medication, bathing and grooming. With limited time per visit, companionship was an ancillary duty. Cordial conversations took place between the care workers and the home care recipients, but the short duration of the visits meant that these conversations were quick and often job related. Paramedical care such as wound dressing and administering injections cannot be carried out by the home care workers in Denmark and is the responsibility of the domiciliary care nurse. The domiciliary care nurse was present twice during a home visit, and the relationship between the care worker and the nurse seemed to be cooperative and professional. 'Free choice', whereby the care recipient indicates that they would like the care worker to do alternative care tasks, was not evident in any of the visits. One home care recipient queried whether the home care worker could rearrange some furniture, but the home care worker indicated this was not within the remit of her job.

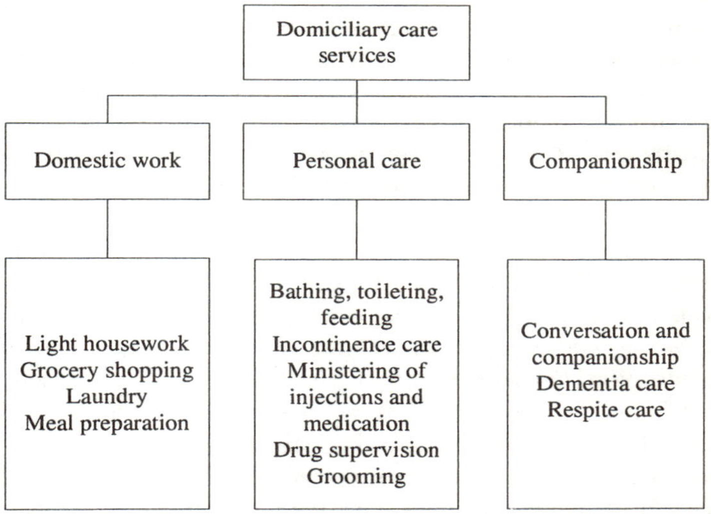

Figure 6.1 Duties of a home care worker

As mentioned above, Cleo in San Francisco jokingly described her job as being similar to a nurse's job in a nursing home, but on a lower salary. Cleo typically delivers both domestic and personal care. Companionship care is also an important and accepted element of the job. Cleo's visits typically last from one and a half to three hours, so tasks such as cooking can be done slowly and under the instruction of her client. When caring for her mother, she explained that she was paid for 80 minutes a day, and even if her mother could not find chores for her to do, she explained that she would always think of something to do. Stacy, the IHSS care recipient, outlined how she likes to train her care workers to administer personal care and likes to show them how to cook and prepare specialist cuisine.

While the work of a domiciliary care nurse is not comparable to the work of an unskilled domiciliary care worker, it was insightful to see the broad range of medical services that Hilda the home care nurse delivered in the home in Germany. The majority of her clients could be classified as 'high-dependency' clients who required regular paramedical assistance. While companionship is not a duty of a domiciliary care nurse, Hilda, a warm and effervescent individual, affectionately greeted each of her clients with a hug. Despite the shortness of the visits, she conversed with the clients in a friendly and companionable manner and also sat down with one client to have their daily cigarette break together.

Marie, the German domiciliary care worker, also seemed to have a very close, informal and cordial relationship with both of her clients. In contrast to Hilda's brief visits, Marie had one hour per visit. Like Helena in Denmark, Marie worked in a dual capacity, delivering both personal and domestic care. Food shopping for clients was a regular duty of Marie's, whereas this usually was not the case for Helena in Denmark, as private companies had entered the market, providing a food shopping service for persons in need of such assistance. Marie also did light housework chores and delivered personal care such as bathing and changing incontinence pads.

Home Environment

Observing the different home settings – from the white cosy porta-cabin with the fire blazing in Germany to the old but welcoming apartment in Denmark with family photos displaying proudly the chronicles of life on the walls, to the apartment in San Francisco where all belongings were stored away in an ordered neat fashion – brought home the intrinsic worth of domiciliary care. While the home setting may not be the preferred choice of all long-term care recipients, the option of staying in one's familiar environment, complete with the trinkets and memorabilia collected over a lifetime should be available to all who desire it. Arguably, the ability to remain at home preserves the independence and autonomy of older people and enables couples with severe care needs to remain living at home together. For example, the above-mentioned scenario in Denmark of the 90-year-old woman supervising the care of her husband would be difficult, perhaps impossible, in the confines of a nursing home.

The intimacy and uniqueness of the care relationship in the home is apparent when observing such work. The one-on-one relationship between a care worker and a home care recipient is a complex one: trust, sensitivity, compassion, efficiency, respect, humour and warmth are all required at different times according to the particular care needs of the individual. While technical competencies are obviously essential, the important social component of care should not be overlooked.

Cultural issues relating to 'care in place' became apparent during the observation exercises. In Denmark, the bedroom of the ethnic minority woman with multiple health problems was more akin to a hospital room than a bedroom. Her family did not want her to enter institutional care, as this would reflect badly on them, yet ironically it seemed, in the care worker's opinion they could not provide her with the intensive care she required. Obviously, in this instance the wishes of the family need to be recognised, yet the question must be posed whether there is a limit to how hospital-like the home can become and whether there are certain instances where the resources (including provision of informal care) in the home are not sufficiently adequate to ensure the continued delivery of intensive domiciliary care.

In Germany and Denmark, it was clear that some of the care recipients that Hilda and Helena visited had no social contact outside of their visits. This was particularly worrisome for one such recipient in Denmark and one in Germany, each of whom suffered considerable ill health and lived alone. In both cases, the care recipients lived in old, dark and musty accommodation and it was difficult to imagine how they managed on a day-to-day basis. In such poor living conditions it seems pertinent to ask whether care in an alternative setting offering more scope for social interaction would be preferable.

Monitoring and Support of the Home Care Worker

Monitoring of and auxiliary support for care workers seemed to be better developed in Germany and Denmark than in California. In Germany and Denmark, the home care workers were issued daily with time sheets and forms, which they had to complete and return. In Denmark, two meetings of care workers were held daily, the first to outline the day's agenda and the second to discuss any concerns about clients they had visited during the day. The provision of such a debriefing exercise and the subsequent professional support may be viewed as a distinct advantage of the Danish system, as observed during the observation exercise, although whether this practice occurs universally across Denmark or is a unique feature of this public sector organisation is unknown. In contrast to this supportive environment, the home care workers in San Francisco's IHSS programme seemed to be offered little professional support and had little or no contact with the PA.

In both Germany and Denmark, clients were periodically rotated, regardless of whether this was in accordance with the preferences of the home care recipients. Helena, the home care worker in Denmark, explained that, in her opinion, it is essential that particularly intensive clients be rotated. The issue of safety was raised in Germany and San Francisco. In Germany, Hilda explained how one client had threatened to hit her a number of times. Because of the instability of this client, care workers are regularly rotated, and not expected to care for him for prolonged periods. Furthermore, in the case of particularly demanding clients in both Germany and Denmark, two care workers will sometimes be present; this option is not available in the IP mode in the IHSS. In San Francisco, Cleo explained how a male client had sexually harassed her and she promptly quit the job, since she did not see any other recourse, 'Who do you go to when he does that? Who do you tell? So I left and let him get somebody else'.

Time

Closely related to the quality of the care relationship is the amount of time that a care worker can spend with a care recipient. Of the three domiciliary care observation exercises, time was most restricted in the Danish case, with visits typically lasting 20 minutes, and not going beyond 30 minutes. In Germany, the home care worker spent one hour with each client, while in San Francisco the time spent with the client varied according to their needs, but typically lasted 80 to 120 minutes.

While the IHSS care worker in San Francisco delivered care to only three care recipients, the care worker in Denmark sometimes provided care to as many as ten people daily. In Germany, the domiciliary care worker usually visited five care recipients daily, while the domiciliary care nurse visited as many as 22 in an average day.

The difficulty of strictly abiding by specified time allotments was apparent in both Denmark and Germany. In both cases, weather conditions were bad. Not only did wet clothes have to removed upon entry to a house and be put back on when exiting the house, but snow and frost meant that cycling, walking and driving was at times difficult. No allowance is made for these hazardous conditions and home care workers must endeavour to complete their work in the prescribed time.

In Denmark, following the introduction of 'free choice', the care recipient is able to direct the work of the domiciliary care worker. However, the ability to do this to the extent that the recipient requires seems difficult within the limited time allocated. Allotment of time in the IP contract mode in San Francisco is determined by the home care recipients and as such grants the care recipients greater levels of control over the care they receive. Stacy, the IHSS home care recipient, had 171.3 hours per month (approximately five hours a day) to divide among her three home care workers. While it is unwise to generalise on the basis of a small number of observation meetings, it would seem that the ability to foster more companionable friendships is most likely in the IHSS system where care workers can visit for two to three hours at a time. The close relationship that develops as a consequence of these relatively lengthy visits was evident in Cleo's case. She explained that she would visit a client in hospital, even though she would not get paid for doing so. Furthermore, in San Francisco, time allocation is flexible and dictated by the home care recipient rather than the home care organisation, which, arguably, places the home care recipient in a more powerful position.

The amount of time the care worker is allocated has a significant impact on the level of social interaction that can take place between the care worker and the home care recipient. In addition, the level of social interaction seemed to be closely associated with the level of dependency of the care recipient. Considerably less conversation and interaction took place between care workers and home care recipients with high-dependency needs than care recipients with low-dependency needs. Moreover, the exchange between the home care worker and the care recipient can often be a consequence of the personality dynamics between them. Thus, differences in engagement levels can frequently be a function of personalities, with some care recipients seeming to prefer a more distanced 'non-intrusive' professional relationship than others, who no doubt favour a more 'personalised' approach and look forward to their daily visit and conversation with their domiciliary care worker. While the home care workers in all cases were warm and friendly, the heavy workload, particularly of Helena in Denmark, meant that she had to approach her job with an air of efficiency and functionality in order to get the necessary tasks done in the allocated time. As outlined in Chapter 3, there has been a noticeable rationing of care time awarded in recent years in Denmark particularly to low dependency persons, and, indeed, the effects of such rationing were apparent in the Danish observation exercise.

Informal Caregiving

The three observation exercises were of formal domiciliary care workers. The complex world of familial caregiving was not directly explored in this study. Within the observation exercise in Denmark, familial caregiving was not very evident. The non-Danish home care recipient mentioned above was receiving intensive domiciliary personal care (up to six visits a day) on the premise that the family would supply adequate domestic care, but this was deemed to be an exception rather than the rule by the domiciliary care worker. In Germany, familial care was more apparent, and in one instance a family caregiver was present. Also, in Germany, Hilda reiterated that all of the clients she visited that day were housebound due to the bad weather conditions and, in one way or another, were dependent on their family to help out. Hilda also stated that in her opinion some of the care recipients that she visits are neglected by their family (indeed, one such case was outlined above), and that the doctor will not take action and advise them to get professional services. She believed that many family members are forced to look after parents because the cost of domiciliary care has risen considerably and people have to 'spend down' their money before they will be entitled to free social care or nursing services. In California, Cleo the home care worker explained how she had taken care of her mother, bathing and delivering personal care, and pointed out that she would not have had it any other way. Stacy, the home care recipient in California, also explained how her mother had the dual responsibility of caring for her and her father, who had a disability, before she was awarded additional care benefits through the IHSS programme.

CONCLUSIONS

An understanding of how the domiciliary care work functions on the ground is essential when analysing a care regime. As Twigg (2000, p. 1) comments, 'It is at the front line that the true nature of care reveals itself. It is there that it is created; and only there can it be judged'. While it is obviously impossible to fully characterise the multifaceted worlds of home care by means of short observation exercises, these exercises proved informative. The most significant commonality between the three contexts was that in each case, the care workers operate in a dual capacity, providing both personal and domestic care. Apart from this, the practices varied considerably, with the most significant difference possibly relating to the amount of time available to deliver care tasks: the shorter 'bursts' in which care was delivered in the Danish and German contexts contrasted markedly with the lengthy stretches of care awarded in the US context. From the care worker perspective, the arrangement observed in the US offers less support and job security than the German and Danish arrangements, yet it does appear to permit greater levels of flexibility and, in some instances, arguably, facilitates a closer relationship between the care worker and care recipient.

The amount of time awarded to a care recipient has fundamental implications for the care relationship and the quality of care delivered. If home care is viewed as a care service similar to that provided in a nursing home, the emphasis is on care that is delivered efficiently and in accordance with quality standards: the domiciliary care worker goes in, is polite, does the work well and departs for the next client. In a model where time is not as rationed or limited, the opportunity for companionship, discussion and the fostering of a stronger interpersonal relationship is nurtured. The advantages and disadvantages of each type of relationship, as seen from the care recipients' perspective, is an important issue, which has enormous implications for levels of satisfaction with the service they receive. This is something that was not adequately explored in the current study but which requires further investigation.

In all three contexts provisions were in place to ensure that care delivery is of a high standard. However, the extent and nature of these provisions varied widely. Naturally, the notion of quality varies depending on the perspective from which it is advanced (that is, administrators, home care recipients, family members or care workers). Within this study it was not possible to explore 'quality' adequately. Furthermore, quality issues may differ according to the age, dependency level and needs of the individual. Suffice it to say that the responsibility of the care recipient for ensuring quality is considerably higher in the US context than in the two European contexts, especially in the case of the IP mode which, arguably, brings into close relief the potential clash between freedom and flexibility, on the one hand, and security and responsibility, on the other.

NOTE

1. There may be problems with the reliability and generalisability of observational data. Findings may reflect only a small sample of the population and, therefore, cannot be generalised to others. There is also the possibility of observer effects (where observation may distort the behaviour of those observed).

7. Comparing Domiciliary Care Policies: Similarities, Differences and Innovations

Chapters 3, 4 and 5 reviewed key aspects of the domiciliary care systems in Denmark, California (USA) and Germany in detail. Chapter 6 approached the subject from a different perspective by drawing on observation and interview data to provide an insight into domiciliary care services as they operate 'on the ground'. Taking into consideration the findings of these four chapters, an attempt will now be made to amalgamate this information. Particular areas of divergence and convergence in the three systems will be noted, together with how these relate to current comparative discussions on social care systems. With this in mind, Chapter 7 has been divided into seven themes:

1. the eligibility criteria employed within each system;
2. the comparative differences of the regulatory and administrative systems of the respective care regimes;
3. the comparative differences of their financial systems;
4. the arrangements for the delivery of care services, the introduction of social care markets and provider pluralism in the service provider mix;
5. workforce issues and the recommodification of the care labour force;
6. the varying degrees of consumer power granted to care recipients in each social care regime; and
7. the degree to which the state formally promotes familial care (by paying family caregivers).

Returning to the notion of welfare state typologies and social care paradigms, as discussed in Chapter 1, the Danish system can be categorised as 'statist' (where the state takes extensive responsibility), the US as part of the familial/individualist model (where families and individuals are responsible for financing and delivering the bulk of care), and Germany as belonging to the 'state pays, others provide' paradigm, where the state has expanded its role in financing care, that is, overwhelmingly provided by families but also by not-for-profit (and, increasingly, private sector) organisations (see Timonen, 2005). While these labels may broadly encapsulate some of the central characteristics of the systems, in reality, all countries have 'mixed' regimes that are constantly evolving. As the discussion below will elucidate, new trends such as the introduction of social care markets, the increasing reliance on informal care and the new role of intermediary organisations are causing the distinctions between these typologies to become less clear-cut.

Within the three countries the provision and financing of domiciliary care has traditionally taken three forms, namely: (i) services in kind (the predominant mode in Denmark); (ii) cash allowances with restrictions (the predominant mode in Germany, where long-term care insurance (LTCI) benefits are used to purchase care from formal providers and to reward family caregivers; in the US the In-Home Supportive Services (IHSS) also fall under this heading) and (iii) 'personal budgets' whereby eligible individuals are awarded money that enables them to purchase services as they see fit. The third option is being discussed in Germany, piloted in Denmark and available in parts of the US (although not through the IHSS programme in California). We shall discuss each in turn, starting with the way in which eligibility to care is determined.

ELIGIBILITY FOR HOME CARE

The procedures that are used to determine eligibility for home care vary considerably between the three countries reviewed (Table 7.1). Denmark can be viewed as having the most egalitarian eligibility system, with universal eligibility extended to all Danish citizens in need of care in their home: financial background or means are not taken into consideration in the eligibility assessment. The eligibility assessment is conducted by a nurse employed by the municipality and is not based on either strict functional capacity or specified minimum standards. Instead the eligibility assessment is based on a holistic approach, with the psychosocial aspects of potential care recipients' lifestyle and their needs and circumstances taken into consideration. A preventive home care visit (or eligibility visit) is offered twice a year to all persons over 75 years of age. The use of such preventive visits de-stigmatises the notion of additional care in the home and ensures that home care services are delivered efficiently and in a timely manner before a person's condition starts to deteriorate.

As in Denmark, Germany's LTCI system covers everyone and does not take into account financial resources. However, benefits are provided only to those meeting fairly strict functional status criteria. In this assessment, functional ability is divided into three levels of care need, which differ according to the number of difficulties with activities of daily living (ADL); beneficiaries are thus classified as having substantial, severe or very severe care needs. A national standardised assessment ensures that equity (based on functional ability) is guaranteed. A nurse employed by the insurance funds conducts the eligibility assessment. The eligibility tool measures primarily the applicant's physical capacity.

Table 7.1 Central features, qualifying conditions and assessment in the three home care contexts

	Denmark: (public) long-term care	California: IHSS	Germany: LTCI
Coverage/ eligibility	Universal	Means-tested	Universal
Approximate number of domiciliary care beneficiaries	206,886[a]	283,750[b]	Approx. 1.38 million[c]
Qualifying conditions and assessment	Individual needs assessment Assessment carried out by care evaluator (qualified nurse) who is a municipal employee Some consideration is given to the presence of a healthy spouse within the household	Assessment based on need for help in ADL, assessed with the help of a state-issued assessment form County-based social workers conduct assessments Available help such as that provided by a spouse is considered	Universal assessment based on functional ability – three levels of disability. Threshold for obtaining benefits is limitations in two ADLs and a need for help in some IADLs Assessment conducted by physicians employed by Medical Offices of the Sickness Funds No account taken of household situation or financial means

Sources: [a] Statistics Denmark 2006; [b] Data from 2002 (Kitchener et al., 2002) ; [c] Data from 2004, excludes LTCI beneficiaries accessing institutional care (Federal Ministry of Health).

In stark contrast to the two European countries, eligibility for publicly financed domiciliary care services in the United States is means-tested and restricted to a small section of the US population. Commenting on the provision of publicly financed domiciliary care in the United States, Feder (1999, p. 4) states cynically: 'In long term care, there is no system; almost nobody has protection' (see also Feder et al., 2000). In California persons receiving social welfare benefits or supplementary security income (SSI) are financially eligible for IHSS services, provided that the value of their liquid assets also falls below a stated maximum value. Persons who have an income greater than SSI monthly payments make co-payments or 'cover their share of costs'. Like in Germany, a state-wide uniform assessment tool is used to measure functional status.

A central goal of any domiciliary care system should be that parity and equal access to services are guaranteed. The use of a national eligibility tool and the enforcement of strict national assessment protocols is one way of ensuring a more objective assessment. However, universal assessment tools can also unwittingly disadvantage certain groups who require specialist care. For example, Germany's LTCI assessment tool has been criticised for discriminating against some groups such as those with cognitive difficulties. It does not, for example, adequately measure the need for supervision of such groups. However, with the recent development of a specially adapted assessment tool for persons with cognitive difficulties such as dementia, some progress has been made to address this. In the US some of those interviewed for the purposes of the research suggested that in spite of the use of a uniform assessment tool, some discrepancies still exist between the counties as to how the instrument is administered and as such state-wide parity is not always guaranteed.

REGULATORY STRUCTURES

There are significant discrepancies between the regulatory environments of the three care systems reviewed (Table 7.2). The key differences concern the level at which the programmes are administered and the balance of responsibility between central government, local government and service users. In Denmark and the United States, regionalisation (or responsibility at local government level) of service provision is important. In both instances, the broad legal framework is specified by the central/federal government, while responsibility for how the home care service 'programme' is delivered, supervised and regulated is decided by the local government. As a result, the extent to which a municipality in Denmark, or a state in the United States, channels its resources and finances into its domiciliary care system is influenced more by the priorities of the respective state/municipality administrators than in Germany.

An explicit goal of Danish social care policy for older people is to prevent institutionalisation, by assisting older people to help themselves within their home (or assisted living dwelling). Local politicians in the Danish municipalities determine the social services budget and the amount of money they will channel into the domiciliary care services budget on an annual basis. They also have to ensure that there is an adequate supply of services, that preventive home call visits are conducted and that adequate quality assurance mechanisms are in place. Electoral mechanisms within Denmark ensure that the public can continually put pressure on elected administrators to provide high-quality domiciliary care services. As in other countries, the fact that a growing proportion of the Danish electorate is aged 65 or over means that, increasingly, this cohort will be an important political pressure group, something which arguably should translate into a continued supply of adequate care services.

Table 7.2 Quality controls in the three home care contexts

	Denmark: (public) long-term care	California: IHSS	Germany: LTCI
Legislation, general control and oversight	General guidelines from central government, implementation and detailed provisions by local government	Relatively little guidance and control from central government	Strong guidance and control from central government
Quality assurance	Quality guidelines are outlined on an annual basis by the local government. These can vary substantially between municipalities – in some areas they include stipulations on minimum criteria for formal service providers	Providers operating under the agency contract mode follow strict quality and monitoring controls. Care recipients under the IP mode are visited once a year by social workers, so that quality assurance is heavily reliant on the feedback of home care recipients	Recipients of cash benefits are visited by a nurse employed by the care insurance funds every three or six months depending on level of care. Owners and managers of domiciliary agencies are required to develop guidelines for assuring quality service

In recent years, however, there has been a reorganisation of the Danish domiciliary care system. The most notable feature of this reorganisation has been the delineation of the role of the municipality as the supplier and regulator of home care services. This reorganisation coincides with an emerging trend in

Denmark towards a more nationally regulated system, which ensures greater transparency and permits easier cross-municipal comparisons. By streamlining (or dichotomising) the responsibility of the municipality, it has been argued that the federal government is in a better position to coordinate, regulate and monitor service delivery and perhaps most importantly to track spending. As a result, the local government still retains most of the regulatory and administrative powers (and undoubtedly will continue to do so), and new levels of monitoring and supervision of the domiciliary care systems at the national level have increased.

Germany's long-term care system, in contrast, is largely centralised with responsibility for regulation entrusted to the insurance funds. The extensive and complex legal guidelines specified by the federal government for the delivery of the LTCI insurance programme are nationally applicable. Prior to the introduction of an LTCI scheme, the federal states, or *Länder*, had the main responsibility for the provision of long-term care services within their jurisdiction. However, with the introduction of the LTCI Act, this responsibility was passed on to the insurance funds. The insurance funds are bound by detailed federal legislation, which is strictly enforced and deals with eligibility assessment, supervision, service delivery, the value of care awarded and quality assurance. Fundamental to this legislation is that equity and parity are guaranteed throughout Germany. The legislation is specified by the federal government and the *Länder* have little control over the insurance funds. Nevertheless, the local government (*Länder*) still have significant power to shape and influence national legislation in the area of long-term care by approving or vetoing any changes to the legislation that the federal government wants to introduce. In contrast to Denmark, however, political influence from the over-65 population on the development of the LTCI is not as visible. As Alber (1995, p. 137) points, out 'only economically active contributors, but not pensioners are represented in the funds [administrative boards]', which may be one explanation why 'cost containment interests predominate over need satisfaction interests'.

Provision of home care services in the US is largely decentralised. Campbell and Morgan (2005, p. 12) point out that in the US 'there is greater independence between levels of government and, thus, a tendency by policy makers to shift burdens around rather than confront their underlying cause'. For this reason, there are huge disparities across the US in: (i) the provision, availability and entitlement to publicly funded social care services and (ii) the emphasis placed on institutional care compared to domiciliary care. The only obligatory programme that all US states are authorised to provide is the home health programme, whereby care is provided for a short duration or for a period of acute need. At their own discretion, states can provide waiver programmes or a state-plan personal care programme.

State-plan personal care programmes, as the name suggests, are administered at the state level and as a means-tested entitlement programme must be available throughout the state if they are made available at all. While the state provides almost half of the financing for these programmes, regulation and administration of the programme is at the county level. For this reason, the delivery of this programme can vary substantially across the various counties. In California, for example, variations such as the existence of the agency contract mode, the make-up of the PA board and the wages and social security benefits of care workers are all determined at county level. As a result, efforts by counties to contain costs can influence the regulation, administration and delivery of the programme. Pressure or consumer groups with the most political influence have tended to be those associated with the disability movement as opposed to older service users. Wiener and Stevenson (1998) state that while elderly advocacy groups are well organised and financed in some states such as New York and Wisconsin, this is not the case for other states such as Alabama and Mississippi. Furthermore, because services in the US are residual and means-tested, a greater emphasis is placed on individual responsibility through private insurance, informal care or individual purchase of formal or 'grey' market care.

The role of intermediary organisations and the establishment or strengthening of local partnerships or community not-for-profit support groups is another important influence emerging in the three domiciliary care systems. The importance of such organisations was raised in the interviews in Germany, with key policy officials referring to the need for an increased emphasis on community activity and delivery of low-threshold activities for older people. However, the fact that the *Länder* are not legally obliged to provide such ancillary community support programmes means that in most instances the authorities renege on this duty. In Denmark the long tradition of public service provision has meant that, traditionally, activity in the voluntary sector was not very visible. However, the Danish central government has begun to recognise the important niche this sector could provide, and since 1996 has allocated finances to voluntary organisations working to strengthen the support networks of older people. It is difficult to know whether the activities of these intermediary organisations will have any fundamental impact on the delivery of social services or bypass the role of the local authorities. However, it seems highly probable that with predicted rises in the number of older people in each of the three countries the role of these organisations is likely to increase and perhaps become an integral aspect of the respective long-term care systems.

FINANCING STRUCTURES

In Denmark home care is financed by general tax revenue, both local and national. Similarly, in the US, state-plan personal care programmes are jointly funded by local and national taxes. In Germany home care is financed through a mandatory insurance scheme (see Table 7.3). There is, however, a key difference between the US and Danish financing systems, in that within Denmark fiscal equalising programmes ensure that poorer or less economically advantaged municipalities are provided with financial assistance. In the US, however, this is not the case. As Campbell and Morgan (2005, p. 12) write, 'the United States has never adopted the kinds of fiscal equalizing programs used in other federal systems. There is no common pool of tax dollars so that increased burden in some states will impinge on the fiscal health of others'.

Table 7.3 Central features of the financing structure within the three home care systems

	Denmark: (public) long-term care	California: IHSS	Germany: LTCI
Central features of financing	Financed through local and national tax revenue, using equalising mechanisms between local governments	Financed through local and national tax revenue, does not use significant equalising mechanisms. Emphasis on cost control	Financed through employee and employer social insurance contributions. These, as well as the benefit levels, have been capped since 1994

This means that in the US (unlike Denmark) country/state financial capacity can dictate the amount of services available. According to Alber (1995), programmes that receive joint funding from both local and central governments tend to facilitate an expansion of services, presumably because there is a greater of pool of money available. However, he also notes that 'each level of government then has an interest to shift the burden of financing to the other, while preserving as much autonomy from regulation as possible' (p. 146).

Across the three countries efforts to contain spending on long-term care can be identified at both national and local levels. For example, in the US there are caps on the extent to which the federal and state governments will subsidise the wages of care workers as well as the overall budget; in Denmark there have been notable decreases in the amount of care awarded, which is thought to coincide with a new emphasis on controlling costs; while in Germany, caps are placed on the value of care awarded, and the fact that the value of payments has not changed since the inception of the programme is likely to reflect that an important emphasis is placed on cost control.

Wiener and Stevenson (1998) outline a number of strategies which US states have utilised to curtail spending on long-term care programmes. These include: (i) encouraging private LTCI and a clampdown on persons transferring their assets to access the Medicaid programme; (ii) integrating acute and long-term care services; (iii) using traditional cost-control mechanisms such as limiting expenditure per person; (iv) controlling the supply of providers and (v) cutting reimbursement rates. Meijer et al. (2000) also offer an interesting commentary on how financial savings are made in Germany and Denmark (as well as in Belgium and the Netherlands) on institutional care. They argue that cost savings are made by: (i) extending co-payments; (ii) encouraging cheaper forms of care and (iii) putting pressure on nursing homes to operate at lower costs.

In one way or another, all of the above were found to be important factors in the contexts studied. User fees are required in both Germany and California (for those with incomes over the SSI benefit), while limiting per person spending was mentioned in Germany, Denmark and the US. The use of waiting lists and enforcement of stricter eligibility assessments was alluded to in interviews in the US. Similarly, stricter time-monitoring and the rationing of care awarded was said to have occurred in all three countries due to fears of overspending. The targeting of services to higher-dependency care recipients was found to be evident in both the US and Denmark. To varying degrees, both countries have had to focus services on persons with extensive (personal care) needs and to make some cuts in respect of domestic duties (for example, the IHSS allocates a maximum monthly number of hours to domestic chores). Another cost-saving mechanism, that is, the use of lower-skilled workers, which translate into cheaper labour costs, was also referred to in interviews in all three countries.

It is useful to analyse the financing of domiciliary care within a more general framework that includes the provision and funding of public residential nursing home care. Since 1987, Denmark has operated a system in which community care has been strongly prioritised over institutional care and, indeed, considerable fiscal savings have been made as a result of this new reorganisation. No such policy directives have been taken in either the US or Germany. In fact, the number of people in residential care seems to have increased in both the US and Germany over the past ten years. For example, Stuart and Weinrich (2001) point out that while the number of nursing home beds fell by 30 per cent between 1985 and 1997 in Denmark, it increased by 12 per cent in the United States. One factor that can influence resource allocation and subsequent investment in the home care sector as opposed to the residential nursing home sector is the political landscape and power of the nursing home industry. As Wiener and Stevenson (1998, p. 96) explain, the for-profit nursing home care providers in the US 'are frequent and large contributors to the political campaigns of governors and state legislators' and are the strongest lobby group with regard to the Medicaid programme in the US. Similarly, Kitchener and Harrington (2004, p. 97) who offer an insightful discussion on the historical development of nursing home and community care developments in the US, concluded that 'the relative power and organization of the consumer and nursing home lobby is a key factor' in relation to the development of home and community-based services in the five states they analysed. In Denmark, in contrast, nursing homes are largely run by the municipality and operate on a not-for-profit basis, while in Germany, 26 per cent operate on a for-profit basis, 49 per cent are not-for-profit and 25 per cent are public (Meijer et al., 2000). This would suggest that in these two countries lobbying from the private sector is less pronounced.

While all three systems confront financial challenges, Germany has some unique fiscal concerns due to the fact that the programme essentially operates as a pay-as-you-go programme. In Germany, the fact that neither the mandatory insurance contribution rate nor the value of service tasks contracted out have increased, means that the purchasing power of the LTCI funding is decreasing. In addition, Germany's reliance on the fact that people are more likely to take the cash as opposed to the benefit option has been viewed as a potential weakness for the viability of the LTCI system. It is likely that there will be a higher demand for direct service provision as the availability of family support decreases (as a result of an increase in female labour market participation and a decrease in the birth rate); the implications are that this may cause considerable fiscal pressure, which, in turn, could threaten the sustainability of the system. Furthermore, there is a concern that the projected increase in the number of people with dementia, who require more intensive care and supervision, will also put an additional financial burden on the programme. However, policy makers and politicians alike are cognisant of these weaknesses and are beginning to discuss possible ways of averting the funding crisis.

Finally, successfully integrating long-term care services and acute (health) care services (and related rehabilitation services) has been argued to result in better quality care and cost savings (Wiener and Stevenson, 1998; Merlis, 2000). Germany has not succeeded in negotiating this overlap of acute and long-term care well with cost-shifting exercises taking place among the sickness and LTCI funds. Germany's LTCI programme is administered by the same sickness funds that award care to those with acute care needs, but the budgets for acute and long-term care remain separate. As pointed out in Chapter 5, incentives exist for the LTCI funds to shift potentially costly clients into the sickness insurance scheme and vice versa. As a result of this, opportunities are missed to better integrate long-term and acute care services. Similarly, in the US many states have failed in this regard, with some Medicaid programmes seeking to maximise clients' use of Medicare home health benefits and hence reduce Medicaid costs.[1]

Denmark, in contrast, has adopted an interesting solution to the integration of services. Provision of long-term care and acute hospital care is the responsibility of the municipality. Furthermore, a municipality is penalised if a patient has to remain in hospital after a specified discharge date and must pay another municipality if the necessary services are not available in their own jurisdiction, thus creating a powerful (financial) incentive to ensure that adequate long-term care services are made available immediately following discharge from a hospital. The benefits of coordinating long-term care and acute care are contested. While integrated services are advantageous, there is a view that the integration of acute and long-term care services is not practical. Some critics argue that an amalgamation of acute and long-term care services could lead to the neglect of the long-term care service, the prioritisation of acute over long-term care needs and the 'medicalisation' of long-term care (see Wiener and Stevenson, 1998; Brodsky et al., 2000). None the less, it is important that care systems do not jeopardise the delivery of adequate acute and long-term care and that a separation of these does not compromise the delivery of either.

DELIVERY STRUCTURES

The notion of welfare pluralism or welfare mix has been developed to encapsulate the fact that a wide range of actors across the public, private and voluntary sectors are involved in the provision and financing of care services (see, for instance, Evers and Svetlik, 1993). It appears that an increasingly prevalent element of this mix is the introduction and expansion of market principles, as noted by numerous researchers conducting comparative analysis research on welfare and social care systems (O'Brien and Penna, 1998; Kröger, 2001; Lethbridge, 2005). Welfare pluralism was apparent in the current analysis of home care services in Denmark, Germany and the US (Table 7.4).

Table 7.4 Providers of home care within the three home care systems

Denmark: (public) long-term care	California: IHSS	Germany: LTCI
Public sector is the predominant provider, but since 2003 private providers have entered the market and are entitled to compete with public sector providers	The Californian State mandates that IHSS service be provided through the IP mode in all 58 counties, but counties have the option of contracting out care to private agencies. Approximately one-fifth of the counties offer services through both the IP and agency contract modes	Welfare organisations had a privileged position within the social care system, prior to the introduction of LTCI. LTCI funds are, however, required to treat not-for-profit and for-profit organisations equally and to favour them over public agencies

Denmark, a country long associated with provision of services via the public sector, has recently taken steps to expand the care services market. The 2003 'greater choice for the provider' legislation, which separated the municipal regulator from the municipal care service provider, also heralded a new service delivery milieu in which private providers could for the first time compete with public sector providers to offer comprehensive domiciliary care services. While this development has been slow to take off, with many private providers specialising in one or a limited number of tasks (such as domestic care or food shopping), there has been a proliferation of these providers in urban areas.

The insurance funds in Germany are actively encouraged to avail themselves of the services of the for-profit and not-for-profit service providers over public providers. Traditional privileges which were granted to the welfare organisations (reflecting the long-engrained tradition of subsidiarity) by the states prior to 1994 were abolished with the introduction of the LTCI programme. Just over one decade after the introduction of LTCI, almost half of the providers are not-for-profit. According to some of the interviewees in Germany, the LTCI programme has not succeeded in matching provision with demand and the high utilisation of cash benefits is a reflection of this mismatch between demand for and supply of formal services. Furthermore, they argue that service development has not been adequate in some areas, for example, rural localities and small local authorities. In contrast, in other areas there is an oversupply of services due to the unanticipated number of people choosing the cash option.

In California, recipients in the IP mode choose between either an informal contract or a person referred through the PA. While the home care recipient is responsible for the hiring, firing and supervision of the care worker, the county pays the worker directly. Care recipients in the contract mode can in some counties choose between a number of providers to whom the county has contracted out services, or in the case of San Francisco, avail themselves of the services of the Consortium – a not-for-profit organisation, which has secured the contract for San Francisco County. Initially, this not-for-profit organisation competed with for-profit agencies for a share of the county funds, but as it was able to offer superior services and monitoring at a lower cost, it has succeeded in winning the San Francisco County contract for two successive years.

The contracting-out of care and specification of particular service requirements by the funding body (insurance funds, county or municipality) is an important issue. In California, services in the agency contract mode are tendered out. In Denmark and Germany, all providers who offer services within the specified criteria are entitled to offer their services to eligible care recipients. Furthermore, in both Denmark and Germany, providers will be accepted only if they offer their services within a specified price range. In Germany, there is a very small element of flexibility permitted in these price negotiations, while in Denmark one universal price is stipulated for all of the providers in each municipality. Currently, in Germany private for-profit providers tend to be small organisations often with only five to ten staff; the welfare organisations, in contrast, tend to be very large, with hundreds of employees. In Denmark, private providers are new to the market, so as yet it is difficult to surmise whether they will be large or small organisations. The notion of competitive tendering by way of cost stipulations and minimum quality standards can in some instances be problematic and may threaten the viability of some organisations. As Frade and Darmon (2005, p. 113), argue, they may serve as a 'bureaucratic burden' for the small local providers and advantage the larger national providers (in other instances, the inverse of this may actually be true, which seems to be the case in Germany). Competitive tendering by way of cost stipulations may also have an impact on the conditions and social security of the care workforce. For example, in Germany, both for-profit and not-for-profit service providers must employ a qualified nurse to supervise home care workers. To surmount this costly stipulation, unqualified domiciliary care workers are paid a relatively low salary to compensate for the more costly wages of the qualified nurses (this issue is expanded upon in more detail in the next section, on workforce issues).

The introduction of social markets in all three countries is said to encourage competition, improve consumer choice and, consequently, quality of domiciliary care services. In Germany, the notion of 'weeding out the black sheep' was mentioned, in Denmark 'improving competition' was reiterated, while in the US the importance of 'winning the contract from other for-profit providers' was highlighted. The introduction of such markets is said to ensure more efficient delivery of services, encourage competition, improve consumer choice and autonomy and consequent quality of domiciliary care services and enable the public authorities to coordinate and regulate service provision more objectively. Practical issues such as resource constraints, recruitment difficulties and inadequate specialisation of services have also been advanced as causes behind the new trend of outsourcing and privatisation across various welfare states (Bahle, 2003).

The introduction of market mechanisms does not always guarantee subsequent delivery of higher-quality services. Economists, however, might take the opposite view and argue that competition between providers ultimately benefits the consumer (care recipients), because the system allows the consumer to choose and move between providers that they believe offer the best service (see Hirschman, 1970). Under such arrangements, it is assumed that service providers will be forced to offer better-quality and more-competitive services or exit the market. However, with caps on the cost of services in Denmark and Germany, and caps on wages for employees in California under the IP mode, true market dynamics are arguably constrained. In such a market, the service provider landscape is not necessarily dictated by the consumer (leading to the exit of low-quality providers), but instead reflects the number of providers/care workers able to compete within these prespecified budgets and standards.

From the perspective of both the care recipient and the care worker, quality has been found to correspond most closely to the amount of time the care worker is allowed to spend with the client and the ability of the care recipient to direct the work of the care worker (Stack and Provis, 2000; Staehr, 2005). The amount of time allocated to a client and the ability of the care recipient to influence the care duties of care workers is not a reflection of the service provider mix, but an outcome of public financial commitment to the long-term care sector overall, which translates into the amount of time/money awarded to care recipients. The domiciliary care recipient, particularly in California and Denmark, is given leverage to direct the work of the home care worker (which is thought to empower the care recipient and to improve quality of care). However, as is evident from the research, in both Denmark and Germany, budgetary constraints and predefined price arrangements mean that often care workers spend less time with their clients than they would like to. Care tasks are defined in tenths of an hour in California, and often in minutes in both Germany and Denmark. Such rigid time-frames arguably hinder the delivery of high-quality services and are clearly driven by the perceived need to control expenditure.

CARE WORKFORCE ISSUES

The quality of care cannot be separated from the quality of employment in the care services sector and as such a discussion on the care workforce is an important one in any analysis of a country's long-term care system. By its nature, domiciliary care work is atypical: first, the variety of work sites and the intimate setting in which the care work is delivered distinguishes the job from most other professions; second, home care work is predominantly part-time with workers sometimes working only one hour per day; third, split shift work is a common feature of the work, whereby care workers may visit a client in the morning and evening, often quite briefly; and fourth, in many systems the length of tenure of the contract is unpredictable as death, hospitalisation or a new care arrangement mean that an employment contract can cease without notice.

'Recommodification' is a term used to denote an erosion of the standard employer–employee relationship, which can have consequences for an employee's work contract, working times and pay. Recommodification of the labour market means that workers' power and security are decreased while employers' power increases (Esping-Andersen, 1990). The notion of recommodification was important across all three countries and was most noticeable in California (for care workers working under the IP mode) but also visible in both Germany and Denmark. Workers under the IP contract in California are afforded even less job security than a conventional agency home care worker.

Under an IP contract, the home care recipient becomes the care worker's employer and legally can fire the care worker with a minimum of just 24 hours' notice: unless dismissal took place on the basis of obvious discriminatory grounds, the care worker has no legal defence. It must, however, be acknowledged that the introduction of the PA in California has served as a useful mechanism for improving the conditions of care workers, increasing their wages and offering an element of support and improved training.

In Denmark and Germany, the entry of the private sector has, in some instances, introduced a recommodification of the care labour force. In both countries, it was noted that lower-skilled care workers in private agencies are offered least protection and lower rates of pay than their more highly skilled and qualified co-workers in both the private and public sectors. Furthermore, in Germany, care workers employed via the cash benefit option lack the job security typically afforded in the formal labour market. But, they do have entitlement to pension credits and other insurance schemes, which is a major advantage.

The current thinking on the training of care workers is somewhat contradictory and ambiguous in the three countries. On the one hand, Denmark has funded education programmes for older persons wanting to enter the care sector, training for family caregivers is available in Germany, and the PA in San Francisco is attempting to increase the provision of training courses. On the other hand, there is a parallel shift away from the view that training is required. In Denmark, activation of social welfare recipients and a call for the inclusion of more migrant workers has not coincided with a call for training or upskilling of such workers. In Germany, while it is specified that each agency must employ a qualified nurse to work in a supervisory capacity, there are no stipulations on the qualifications of a domiciliary care worker. In California, a dominant view within the PA's governing bodies is that training stipulations for home care recipients are counterproductive. Trade unions offer some protection to the care workforce in Denmark and California. However, as is evident in the case of Denmark, the amount of leverage they have over national policy is limited, as, for instance, in relation to training qualifications.

According to interviewees, there are those within the disability movement who believe that there are advantages to a system that does not enforce minimum training standards. Proponents of this view sometimes argue that non-skilled persons may be better able to deliver companionate and domestic care and that an enforcement of minimum standards could have negative ramifications on the recruitment of domiciliary care workers, which, in turn, could result in a 'bottleneck scenario' with regard to the supply of qualified care personnel. One crucial overarching issue, however, is cost: enforcing minimum training standards is costly. Moreover, the more skilled the care workers, the higher the wages they will demand. The funding of family carers, as practised in all three countries, is also closely related to the issue of training and the subsequent de-professionalising of the care workforce, which is likely to have negative implications for the pay and work conditions of other home care workers. The topic of family care, which also relates to consumer choice, is discussed below.

CONSUMER POWER

The concept of consumer power (Table 7.5) is most ingrained in the US system, with California having the largest consumer-directed programme in the US. Beneficiaries awarded care under the IHSS IP mode in California are granted both consumer choice and direction. They can decide who they would like to employ as their care worker, at what time they would like their care worker to visit and what tasks they would like the care worker to do. Beneficiaries under the agency contract mode are not afforded the luxury of such a flexible care arrangement, but their wishes in relation to 'who and how' are still accommodated as much as possible within the confines of the agency contract mode.

Table 7.5 Consumer choice and direction within the three home care systems

	Denmark: (public) long-term care	California: IHSS	Germany: LTCI
Consumer choice	Care recipients can choose between a public or private provider (although, in some areas, the number of private providers is extremely low)	Care recipients can choose a carer from either their own informal contacts or from a formal list provided by the PA	Care recipients can choose between a cash benefit and direct service delivery. Care recipients who choose the latter option can also choose between a private and not-for-profit provider
Consumer direction	Care recipients can instruct a care worker that they require a different care task than that specified in the care plan. The care worker should oblige but can use his/her own discretion to assess whether the request is reasonable	In the IP mode, the most common care contract, the care recipient hires, fires, directs and supervises the work of the care worker. While there is a formal care plan, the care recipient is given latitude to change this plan as he/she sees fit	Consumer direction for beneficiaries who opt for the cash option is more an outcome of the informal care relationship than a formal mechanism with the LTCI programme. Consumer direction for care recipients who receive care via formal service providers is absent, since care is awarded by task

Employment of a family member	Home care recipients have the right to appoint their own carer to carry out practical care tasks. The municipality subsequently employs the spouse or relative, who is paid the same rate as public domiciliary care workers and is entitled to the same social security benefits. This option, however, is rarely taken up	Within the IP mode, home care recipients can choose a family member to work as their carer. The extent to which this is taken up varies from 29 to 81 per cent across the different counties (Daly et al., 2004)	There is a strong reliance on informal care, and the ability of family members to act as caregivers within the LTCI programme. Informal caregivers are entitled to pension credits and can have special training. Carers who provide at least 14 hours of care a week and have been caring for at least a 12-month period are entitled to four weeks' vacation in the year during which time the insurance funds pay for professional domiciliary care services

Consumer choice in Germany comes in a different guise. For those who choose the benefit-in-kind option, choice is exercised in relation to the service provider; while not as extensive in rural areas, LTCI beneficiaries have a choice among a variety of not-for-profit and for-profit providers. Choice can also be exercised by those who choose the cash option. Those who take this option can choose who they would like to deliver this care, with formal monitoring taking place twice a year for those allocated to care levels 1 and 2, or quarterly for those allocated to care level 3. For this reason, monitoring of care, as in the IHSS system, is largely the responsibility of the LTCI beneficiary. Consumer direction is virtually absent for those who choose the formal delivery option, since care contracts specify care duties, which cannot be changed without the authority of the insurance fund. Consumer direction within the cash option is presumably possible, since the care arrangement is less formal and more flexible.

While cash benefits or self-directed care, as available in California, are not available in Denmark, 'greater choice for the provider' legislation introduced in 2003 has meant that Danish domiciliary care beneficiaries can exercise an element of consumer *direction* hitherto not possible. The introduction of 'free choice' in the Danish legislation means that home care recipients can now direct the work of the home care worker, in so far as they can specify that they require an alternative care duty other than that specified in the care contract. However, there are restrictions as to what the beneficiary can request, and the home care worker ultimately has the final say, as to whether it is reasonable, or practical, to request this alternative task. Consumer *choice* was also encouraged as a consequence of this new legislation, which enables home care recipients to choose between public or private providers. However, this choice is limited in certain areas where there may be only two providers to choose from.

The cash benefit in Germany and the IP mode in California, arguably, offer the most consumer power. Throughout the interviews in all three countries, numerous advantages of the expansion of consumer choice and direction in the respective domiciliary care systems were put forward. Among the advantages listed were: (i) greater autonomy to the home care recipient; (ii) care recipient's ability to decide who will provide him/her with care (that is, family, friend or formal service provider); (iii) encouraging families and neighbours and friends to provide for their ageing relatives/neighbours; (iv) offering employment to family members or friends who may not have been in the workforce; (v) in low-income households the cash benefit boosts the household income; (vi) foreign national citizens can employ caregivers of similar nationality, culture and language; (vii) it enables better delivery of more flexible service (that is, caregiving duties and times can be negotiated) and (viii) from a policy perspective, consumer choice programmes are generally cheaper to run and offer more flexibility in terms of the employment of care workers, which is particularly attractive in the current climate of care staff shortages in the domiciliary care sector.

Disadvantages of consumer choice/direction identified by the interviewees across the three countries included: (i) it is harder to monitor quality and even delivery of care; (ii) it can promote a 'grey' labour care market and precarious employment contracts; (iii) in some instances, greater exploitation of care workers is possible; (iv) it can potentially de-professionalise domiciliary care work and deflate the importance of training and monitoring of care workers; (v) without adequate support and respite, family caregivers can become overburdened; (vi) in the absence of training, adequate quality standards and adequate supervision, a deterioration of health conditions is possible, which can lead to the care recipient requiring more intensive and costly care; (vii) people with mobility problems or cognitive difficulties may not always be able to monitor and supervise and instruct the work of their carer and (viii) it enables the state to take a more distanced 'hands-off' approach: any problems or difficulties that arise may be transferred to the care recipient rather than the state.

Consumer power, as defined by Alber (1995), also relates to the extent that clients are represented on the administrative boards of financing agencies and the degree to which they are able to influence the public providers upon re-election. As noted earlier in the chapter, Danish care recipients hold the most political sway, by way of electing politicians in their municipalities who provide an adequate care infrastructure. In Germany, the voice of the economically inactive over-65 population holds little political power in terms of direct influence, while in California, the extent to which consumer voice/power is encouraged differs between the counties. Some PA advisory boards (such as San Francisco) have a majority of members who are IHSS recipients, which helps to ensure that consumer preferences and demands are heard. Other counties, however, have boards which largely consist of county officials, and in these counties, consumer power/voice is seriously constrained.

FAMILIAL CARE/INFORMAL CARERS

Points (ii–v) under the advantages and point (v) under the disadvantages of consumer choice relate to informal family caregivers. Germany, Denmark and a large proportion of the state-plan personal care programmes in the US allow home care recipients to employ a family member or friend as a carer if they so choose. Of the three systems reviewed, the role and reliance on familial care is arguably most pronounced in Germany. The reasons behind this are largely historical, cultural and socio-political. Delivery of care by family members via the LTCI programme is incentivised, with carers who work more than 14 hours a month being entitled to up to four weeks' 'paid' holiday per year, during which time the LTCI scheme pays for a temporary institutional or other care arrangement. Furthermore, family carers are also entitled to free training courses and receive social security benefits in the form of pensions.

Family care is also of great significance in the IHSS programme. Beneficiaries awarded care under the IP mode are allowed to employ family members as carers. While this practice is believed to be common, exact figures on the number of family caregivers are not available.

While the payment of family caregivers is permitted in Denmark, this option is rarely taken up. It seems probable that the long tradition of public social services and consequent lack of dependency on children are influencing factors in this regard and that the majority of older people are reluctant (and do not want) to ask their children to provide long-term care. As pointed out in Chapter 3, however, research in Denmark has illustrated that the extensive provision of public social care services has not replaced care by family members, but instead has meant that different types of care are transferred between the generations. Recent reorganisation of the Danish home care system and the consequent reduction in the allocation of care hours to low-dependency beneficiaries may mean that increasing amounts of unpaid informal care will be required by those who are not receiving adequate levels of home care (particularly in relation to domestic care).

The extent to which the provision of family care is distributed across different socio-economic groups and between men and women is an important issue. Research in Germany (referred to in Chapter 6) indicates that domiciliary care recipients who avail themselves of the cash option are often less financially secure than those who opt for direct service provision, suggesting that the long-term care payments have the character of an anti-poverty measure and are particularly attractive to women with low earnings potential. Furthermore, in most instances, the majority of such caregivers are middle-aged and often find it difficult to re-enter the labour market once their caregiving duties are over (Groger, 2006).

Wellin (2006, p. 214) argues that the increased reliance on family care within the US state-funded long-term care programmes coincides with an increased emphasis on consumer choice, and the 'misguided cultural idea' that care recipients prefer familial carers and that this care will be of a superior quality. He points out that the continuing success of many consumer-directed programmes, particularly for consumers with high care needs and cognitive impairments, is reliant on the continued participation of family caregivers. Challenging the intentions of this new reliance on familial care, Wellin (p. 213) questions 'whether the rhetoric of consumer choice might obscure a realization of the continued (and now formally sanctioned and compensated) role of family ties in the future care for less affluent families in the US'. He argues that middle-class families can negotiate the best care arrangements, typically by privately purchasing care services, whereas low-income families cannot afford this luxury and are consequently more reliant on family care. Wellin argues that this reinforces existing social inequalities and perpetuates intergenerational poverty. A similar scenario was advanced in relation to the Danish home care system by Lewinter (2004), who argues that supplementary care will be either provided directly by low-income families or purchased privately by higher-income families if the present rationing of home care continues.

CONCLUSIONS

While the three countries can be assigned to existing welfare classifications that broadly relate to the general framework of the countries' respective social protection systems, a number of new trends and similarities are also apparent, which serve to undermine the accuracy of such classifications.

Of the three contexts reviewed, Denmark's domiciliary care system is the most universalistic one, providing services to the largest share of the older population. This is in contrast to both Germany, where services are targeted towards the 'frailest' and financed up to a maximum limit, and the United States, where provision is targeted towards the most financially insecure. The extent of localised or centralised regulation of the three systems varies considerably. In Germany, the LTCI programme is regulated at national level, although the regional *Länder* have a powerful influence over any pertinent legislative changes which could be made and hence can exert some influence. In Denmark, administration of domiciliary care takes place at the local level, although recently there has been a push to improve elements of the regulatory system at national level. In the US, federal states, by comparison with Germany, do not have much leverage over national policy making. State-plan personal care programmes such as the IHSS, receive some funding from the federal level, but are largely administered and regulated at the county and state levels.

There is a noticeable pluralism of providers in the three countries and an opening up of a 'social care market'. In all three, the state has actively promoted the expansion of this care market on the premise that it gives more choice to the consumer and, consequently, improves the quality of service delivered. In California, only a fraction of the eligible care recipients are granted services via a formal service provider. However, where this is available, there generally is a choice of providers. In Germany, beneficiaries who avail themselves of the benefit-in-kind option can choose between a for-profit and a not-for-profit provider. Similarly, in Denmark, all domiciliary care recipients can choose between public and private providers, a significant departure from the traditional Danish welfare state, which suggests a devaluation of the state's role as the supplier of care services.

All three countries have made efforts to control their long-term care spending. However, issues of cost containment and quality improvement are somewhat at odds with each other. While much of the negotiation with the new home care service providers has revolved around cost, the issue of quality is now recognised at the national level in Denmark and Germany with talks on how quality mechanisms can be improved now taking place. However, as service providers are operating with capped budgets, the extent to which service delivery can be improved seems limited. Furthermore, it is highly plausible that a new emphasis on quality without a parallel increase in the amount of money directed towards the service providers may lead to a greater segmentation or recommodification of the home care workforce, where qualifications and training receive less emphasis as a result of an effort to control costs and salaries.

The contribution of family caregivers is being formally recognised in each of the three countries in the form of, for instance, social security benefits awarded to family carers. While employment of family caregivers is permitted under the three programmes reviewed, the extent to which this is taken up in Denmark is limited, although recent trends towards rationing home care services have caused some commentators to speculate that increasing levels of informal care will be required in the future. The viability of the domiciliary long-term care programme, particularly in Germany and California, is arguably dependent on the continued provision of family care. A reduction in family care would have a major impact on demand for formal care and an enormous impact on future long-term care expenditure. The importance of consumer power has been recognised in each of the three domiciliary care systems. As is evident from the discussion in this chapter, multiple arguments can be put forward for the extension or limiting of consumer power. Whatever guise consumer power will take, supervision by the funding body will have to be enforced at some level in order for it to be acceptable to care workers, care recipients and the general public.

NOTE

1. A number of states are, however, attempting to integrate acute care benefits with long-term benefits – such beneficiaries are referred to as 'dual eligibles'.

8. Conclusion: The Future of Domiciliary Care

This study has reviewed the main features of domiciliary care for older people in Denmark, the United States (with an emphasis on the In-Home Supportive Services programme in California) and Germany. In so doing, it has revealed the complexity of both national and subnational care regimes. It has illustrated that the provision of adequate long-term domiciliary care services presents policy challenges for the three countries reviewed and, indeed, for all social care systems. In each of the countries there is now a strong stated policy preference for care in the home as opposed to institutional care, and, increasingly, policies on the ground are bearing out this preference. However, as this book has highlighted, there are considerable differences concerning the level, nature and financing of service provision across the three care systems. In this concluding chapter, five issues that are believed to be important in future discussions on the provision of publicly financed domiciliary care will be discussed: (i) financing and cost control; (ii) the family/state balance; (iii) quality assurance; (iv) the care workforce and (v) the future domiciliary care research agenda.

FINANCING AND COST CONTROL

In the area of financing, a central distinction can be made between insurance and tax-based (including joint funding by the federal and state governments) systems; another salient consideration is whether a programme has to compete for finance with other essential social care services for other groups such as those with HIV or drug-related problems, as this can have an important impact on fluctuations in spending and the sustainability of the programme.

Control of long-term care spending is perceived as an important challenge both at present and in the future in each of the three contexts analysed in this book. Rising long-term care costs have placed increasing pressure on national and local governments to control and monitor long-term care spending. In the light of population ageing, and the perception among some policy makers that cost savings can be achieved through shifting emphasis from institutional to domiciliary care, the channelling of finances into domiciliary care will continue to be of great importance.

Whether eligibility is decided by means- and asset-testing as in the United States, by functional status as in Germany, or by the broader definition of the 'needs of the individual' as in Denmark, has enormous financial implications. Arguably, a universal system of eligibility as in Denmark is an ideal approach, but difficult to attain in low-tax countries such as the United States, and may not be so palatable in strongly familialist care regimes such as Germany's. In contrast to the universalist approach, a residual system such as the one operating in the United States means that thousands of older people just above the income threshold level, and without private insurance, are not eligible for any public assistance. Evers (1995, p. 12), in his discussion on the future financing of long-term care systems in Europe, takes a rather pragmatic approach when hypothesising how fiscal savings may be made in the future:

> All in all, an assessment of the international situation shows that the time has come not only to reconsider traditional concepts and promises, but also to develop criteria for prioritising the allocation of scarce service resources. With this in mind, breaking free from the traditional alternative between residualism and universalism could represent an important new objective. This could, for example, be achieved by a dual system with basic and additional support measures for care service which gives priority to people who live alone and cannot rely on informal caregivers.

As discussed below under the heading 'Family/State Balance', a number of countries such as Belgium and Austria have already begun to take such steps by subsidising the cost of additional private domiciliary care for low-income care recipients.

The tendency of younger, healthy people to underestimate their own risk for the need of long-term care services is reflected by the low number of people who have private LTCI in the United States, a country where publicly funded care services are only available to a minority (see Campbell and Morgan, 2005). This would suggest that countries with expanding older populations cannot assume that the majority of people will take active steps to safeguard their own long-term care needs. Insurance-based systems that are both mandatory and to a significant level funded by the state and/or employers have been successful in creating incentives for (already insured) individuals to purchase supplementary private insurance cover. A large number of countries with very different social care systems (including Germany, Japan, Luxemburg, Austria and the Netherlands) have opted for an insurance-based system of long-term care, where the risk is pooled among the entire population, and private supplementary insurance is available to those who wish to provide extra coverage (for example, in Germany private LTCI can cover accommodation costs, which public LTCI does not cover). The relative success of these programmes in making care more accessible and affordable may serve as an example to other countries that are contemplating the benefits of an insurance-based long-term care system.

There are important fiscal ramifications attached to the level, nature and amount of services that the state is willing to provide or finance. Ideally, long-term care systems would venture beyond the 'curative' approach of caring for the elderly with extensive (personal) care needs. A more ambitious approach would also promote independent living, a healthy diet, social interaction, leisure activities and retention of the skills of older people. However, the general trend tends to be that, instead of widening the remit of home care to cover these 'less essential' aspects, various cost-cutting mechanisms have been introduced to control spending. Reducing the number of care hours awarded or the range of tasks provided (for example, offering fewer domestic care services in order to focus on the provision of personal care), providing token payments to informal caregivers to promote additional 'low-cost' informal care work and opening up the care workforce to a wider group of unskilled care workers are some of the ways the three countries reviewed in this book have attempted to contain costs. While this can be justified on narrow fiscal grounds, there is a serious danger that it could escalate the decline of health and functional abilities for older people. The value of domiciliary care for those with low dependency care needs, if overlooked, may ultimately place a higher strain on more costly services at a later point. Preventive home visit programmes and subsequent delivery of services, targeted at persons with lower care needs (as available in Denmark) have been proven to delay or prevent functional impairment and subsequent nursing home admissions (Stuck et al., 2002).

FAMILY/STATE BALANCE

There are distinct advantages and disadvantages to a system which promotes informal caregiving. The greatest advantage is the amount of autonomy it entrusts to both the care recipient and the informal caregiver. As well as encouraging family support and improving the household budget, family care that is financed or part-financed through the public purse enables some people to choose their preferred caregiver (that is, a spouse, daughter, daughter-in-law and so on). Public funding of care in these instances can only be viewed as promoting the autonomy and rights of the care recipient. Formally recognising the contribution of informal caregivers can also be seen as a sensible move from the point of view of financing care, in the light of the cost savings that are made if the opportunity costs of 'diverting' potential labour market participants to care work are not considered.

Taking a different perspective, it is possible to argue that care delivered by employed caregivers may in some instances be of a lesser duration and quality. Scharlach et al. (forthcoming) who have conducted extensive research in this area found that employed caregivers provided fewer hours than non-employed caregivers and were required to supplement care by relying more on formal care providers, particularly for the delivery of personal care (see also Scharlach et al., 2006). At times the employment of family caregivers can act as a disadvantage to women (the predominant group of caregivers), offering them in some instances (such as Germany) little money, and delaying or preventing their entry into the wider workforce. It can also potentially lead to the development of negative family relations (for overworked caregivers) and contribute to physical and psychological health problems. Unlike paid formal care workers, family caregivers often cannot take a substantial break from their caregiving responsibilities and as such become 24-hour home care workers. Policy makers must be cognisant of these potential negative outcomes and avoid taking family caregiving for granted or treating it as a service that is low cost and has no opportunity costs for carers or society as a whole. The 'low cost' illusion arises from the fact that most family caregivers who receive a cash payment are in practice paid for only a fraction of their services, and 'opportunity costs' are nowhere taken into account.

The early literature on informal caregiving viewed family caregiving in terms of a 'labour of love' and an altruistic desire to help a family member (Lewis, 2000). While this may be the case for many informal caregivers, there is also a cohort of family carers who provide intensive care to family members primarily in order to compensate for the lack of publicly funded care. Perceptions on how much responsibility the state, the individual and the family should have for the care needs of their older citizens/family members in need of assistance vary across countries. The division of responsibility between the state and the family is a controversial issue that research has only partly illuminated. As Daly and Lewis (1998, p. 6) point out: 'we see care as an activity with costs, both financial and emotional which extend across public/private boundaries. The important analytic questions which arise in this regard are how the costs involved are shared, at an individual level and at the more macro level'.

It is sometimes argued that the provision of publicly funded formal care services suppresses the availability of informal care. The OASIS project, a comparative study of urban populations in England, Norway, Germany, Israel and Spain, sought to explore the following hypotheses: (i) whether countries with high levels of social care service provision have low levels of familial care – the 'crowding out' hypothesis – and (ii) the counter-hypothesis of whether high levels of social services provision promote additional familial care – the 'crowding in' hypothesis (Daatland and Lowenstein, 2005, p. 181). The research found little support for either hypothesis and concluded:

> [A] generous welfare state neither reduces nor increases family efforts, but allows the family to re-orient their responsibility towards less burdensome tasks and needs that are poorly covered by services. An increase in service provision will therefore contribute to an increase in the total level of care, and to a more mixed or shared, help profile.

Similarly, research cited in Chapter 3 shows that there is no significant zero-sum relationship between formal and informal care and that informal care is provided in large quantities even in countries such as Denmark that have a very developed formal care system. The key difference was the *type* of care provided: instead of providing round-the-clock heavy-duty care, family members in Denmark were found to offer help in more episodic activities (such as gardening, shopping and transport). As can be seen from the observation exercises recorded in Chapter 6, the Danish domiciliary care system is in many cases able to cater for individuals with extensive care needs. None the less, even in Denmark one or more informal caregivers also typically provide services in tandem with the public services provision.

Informal caregivers returning to the labour market once care duties are no longer required are in a considerably more disadvantaged situation than their co-workers who have not left the labour market. Family-friendly policies in the workplace could help to improve this situation, so that caregivers are allowed to work on flexi-time or part-time contracts for a specified duration. Denmark, for instance, has adopted such policies for those who have a terminally ill family member. However, even if family-friendly policies are introduced, reconciling work and caregiving duties and maintaining a healthy work–life–care balance is still challenging.

Within the three systems reviewed in this analysis, supplementary care, that is, informal care that is provided in addition to care provided or sponsored with public funds, is also essential, especially for persons with extensive care needs. This issue becomes particularly problematic for low-income families, already delivering high amounts of care, who are unable to purchase supplementary private home care. One method of alleviating the excessive informal caregiver burden for this cohort, as used in Belgium and Austria, for instance, is to subsidise the cost of additional private domiciliary care for low-income care recipients. When costs are subsidised in this way, low-income recipients are more likely to receive adequate care and avail themselves of more care from formal service providers. If this practice were introduced in Germany, it could, in some instances, prevent the recourse to institutional care for those with limited financial resources, in addition to relieving some of the pressure on informal caregivers. None the less, it seems that the current trend in many developed countries is for the state to take an 'arm's-length' approach in the provision of care. In such a climate, it seems likely that the state will further distance itself from the responsibility of care provision (and subsequent well-being of the caregiver) and continue to place more of an emphasis on informal care.

QUALITY ASSURANCE

Ensuring that domiciliary care is of high quality is obviously very important given that care work takes place in an environment where the older person is, arguably, more vulnerable than in an institutional environment. However, quality assurance in domiciliary care is also a very complex challenge. Formulation of adequate quality monitoring procedures is made difficult, among other factors, by the perception that budgetary control and concern with quality standards are frequently diametrically opposed. Furthermore, it is hard to guarantee quality (in itself an elusive concept that is open to many interpretations) in the physically dispersed landscape of domiciliary care. Within the three systems studied in this research, the state has distanced itself to varying degrees from the provider role to strengthen its role as a regulator. However, initiatives such as the different manifestations of cash-for-care and the introduction of consumer-directed programmes, such as the IHSS programme in California, have meant that the state is also distancing itself from the monitoring of service delivery. Any problems that arise between the employer (or care recipient) and employee (care workers) in this care contract, can be argued to be more a function of the bad management or judgement of the employer (that is, service user or care recipient), than any action of the state. Furthermore, within this care paradigm, basic training qualifications are rarely enforced. Consumer control, as encouraged within these programmes, does not necessarily equate to an improved service, and the present emphasis placed upon same may serve to neglect a focus on other pertinent quality-related issues. For example, Samuelsson (2000) examined the quality dimensions of home care in Sweden from the perspective of the home care recipient and found that particularly for the 'oldest old', the ability to 'influence' care received was not viewed as an important dimension. Moreover, Samuelsson (p. 199) argues that 'the attributes of continuity, the suitability of personnel and aspects of availability and time are likely to be of increasing importance'.

While the contracting-out of services and the introduction of quasi-market principles have been justified on the grounds of leading to improved quality and choice, this is not necessarily the actual outcome in all instances. The enforcement of quality standards in the cash-for-care and contract-out models is, for the most part, the responsibility of the provider agency and also a consequence of the service-level agreements specified by the state. However, with caps on the amount of money that the state is willing to pay to these providers, it can be argued that the new trend towards outsourcing care has meant that providers are competing on the basis of cost rather than quality. A key factor is how the competitive tendering processes are arranged and whether they favour larger or smaller organisations. For example, in Germany, these stipulations currently serve to advantage smaller providers, while research in Spain and England has shown that such tendering procedures favour larger ones (Frade and Darmon, 2005). Additional consequences of contracting-out care within these narrowly predefined classifications on subsequent quality and delivery of services are still unclear.

Without doubt, the practical, emotional, financial and health implications of keeping individuals with extensive care needs in their home will be the subject of extensive discussion and debate in the coming years. Future generations of older people may have different expectations of the care they should receive. In a world of mass migration and globalisation, older people's preferred modes of care delivery will also need to be investigated and these can clearly be culture as well as country specific. In the realm of domiciliary care, Denmark has been a pioneer, and other countries may come to emulate the emphasis Denmark has placed on assisted living complexes. An increase in assisted living/sheltered housing complexes may well change the long-term care landscape in the future and reduce the number of nursing home residents across many countries. Modern assisted living complexes have many advantages, and as the baby-boom generation enters the care arena, the demand for less-institutionalised care settings is likely to increase as a consequence of both the higher demands and the greater purchasing power of this cohort. Furthermore, these settings may also prove ideal for those who need monitoring and supervision – in particular, people with dementia, an illness that is projected to increase substantially in the coming decades. The planning and structure of these residences, however, demands much forethought, otherwise they may become glorified nursing homes. Ideally, these complexes would cater for both low- and high-dependency clients, and provide adequate ancillary services which promote community participation, activity and a sense of belonging.

THE CARE WORKFORCE

Unfortunately, the debate on long-term care often excludes care workers. The ability of many service providers to contain costs is improved if (lower-skilled) care workers on lower wages are employed. In this climate, the provision of adequate remuneration and social security benefits becomes less of a concern. There is a conflict between professionalising care work, on the one hand, and opening it up to care workers with little or no training, on the other. While a de-emphasis on skills may open up the care workforce (and save money for the state and employers), it also has the negative implications of creating more precarious contracts for care workers and possibly decreasing the quality of services delivered. The difficulty of reconciling consumer choice and workers' rights, particularly in liberal systems such as in the United States, is at times problematic. The state's role in funding these low-paid, low-security jobs is not only contentious but also highly questionable if it leads to the delivery of inferior-quality services.

A number of countries (including Germany, France, the Netherlands and Belgium) have expanded their social care systems in order to both encourage low-wage employment for women and to achieve the goals of their employment policy (Morel, 2006). Morel points out that the absence of clearly defined professional standards and qualifications promotes the creation of low-pay, low-status care jobs for women. She argues that these policies have been veiled in a rhetoric of 'free choice' that tends to mask the fact that this choice is more constrained for low-income families than for economically advantaged families who have the financial ability to purchase private care services. The use of a lower-skilled workforce is a dangerous cost-cutting mechanism in an environment where an increased number of high-dependency clients with co-morbidities and chronic illnesses are requiring care services in the community. As well as requiring basic domestic care, these recipients frequently require substantial amounts of personal care, which, in some instances, can only be delivered by a skilled care worker. Technological advances will no doubt improve the coordination and delivery of these services, but adequate care worker training will be required to ensure that satisfactory care standards are maintained.

The shift from services to cash-for-care in Germany and in some US states has been a significant development that has further downplayed the public sector's role as a provider of services and enhanced its role as the provider of funding. Under this kind of arrangement, the beneficiaries are free to choose who they would like to receive care from, and receive money from the state to reward their chosen carer (albeit, in Germany, this payment is lower where an informal caregiver is chosen). The impact of these new cash-for-care programmes on the changing employment status (and associated social security entitlements) of the home care workers is a topic that remains under-researched. Ungerson (2004) offers a useful introduction to this issue by analysing the cash-for-care schemes in five European countries (Austria, France, Italy, the Netherlands and the United Kingdom) in the context of empowerment of both the care worker and the care recipient. Of the five countries, Austria and Italy had cash-for-care systems that were entirely unregulated. In these countries, in contrast to the other three which had more regulated systems, the money awarded for care was typically incorporated into the generic household budget, used to pay for sporadic caregiving by neighbours or friends, or used to access care workers through the 'grey' market. Caregivers accessed through the 'grey' care market were generally migrant women who had few alternative job prospects. These findings corroborate international research on migrant workers which has indicated that migrant women frequently work in informal and sometimes family-like arrangements, and have precarious work contracts that are not enforceable by law. Rather than leading to an independent status, paid work under these conditions can lead to dependency and vulnerability. Ungerson's findings would suggest that the issue of 'grey' care markets and increasing numbers of migrant workers employed in the elder care sector may be important issues in the coming years if cash-for-care programmes are expanded.

FUTURE COMPARATIVE RESEARCH ON DOMICILIARY CARE

While our study corroborates the value of welfare regimes and social care typologies as heuristic and analytical devices, their usefulness clearly has limits. We observed that an emphasis on the similarities across the three systems helped us to focus better on the key issues within the care systems and enabled us to make a more critical comparative analysis of the advantages and disadvantages of particular care regimes. We found that grouping the care regimes into typologies can often serve to dilute or hide these similarities, which, arguably, may reflect international trends that are more likely to indicate the future direction in which care systems are likely to evolve.

Rather than focusing on the differences which regime classifications tend to highlight, focusing on the similarities enabled us to recognise universal new trends such as: (i) the changing role of the state as a provider and purchaser of services; (ii) the greater acknowledgement of the contribution of informal caregivers; (iii) the requirement that care recipients pay a supplementary fee for additional or ancillary services; (iv) the targeting of services to people with higher-dependency needs and consequent decreased emphasis on domestic care; (v) the recommodification of the care workforce; (vi) the increased focus on consumer power; (vii) the acknowledgment that quality monitoring will become a growing concern in coming years; (viii) a new focus on the value of the voluntary sector and (ix) the exploration of new forms of provision/financing such as the use of personal budgets. Emphasising these similarities also made it easier to examine how different systems tackle similar issues, *inter alia,* the assessment process, rewarding of caregivers, the emphasis placed on institutional care and consumer choice and direction. Therefore, we suggest that future comparative analyses should utilise existing welfare and social care regime classifications but also focus their analysis on new trends which sometimes obey and sometimes contradict these models of social protection and care.

This study provides a number of valuable lessons for researchers conducting comparative analyses of social care, and domiciliary care, in particular. We believe that the framework proposed by Alber (1995) served as a useful analytical tool when comparing the three care regimes. Alber pointed out that social care systems are a result of historical evolution, which reflects, among other things, the church–state and centre–periphery relations and dynamics. To untangle the unique aspects of a care regime, Alber recommends comparing the: (i) 'regulatory'; (ii) 'financial' and (iii) 'delivery systems' of the care regimes and (iv) exploring the extent of 'consumer power'. While Alber originally presented these four aspects of social care regimes as possible explanatory variables, it is clearly also possible to treat them as dependent variables. In this analysis, we have not sought to use them explicitly for explanatory purposes, although our analysis does hint at ways in which the different methods of organising the regulation, financing, delivery and consumer choice influence the 'end product', namely, the extent and nature of care delivered to service users.

The paucity of (comparative) research focusing on domiciliary care on the ground became apparent in the course of this research. While conducting our literature review, we found that there is little research that considers experiences of the domiciliary care system from the perspective of both home care recipients and domiciliary care workers. An understanding of the opinions of both service users and care workers regarding the quality, supervision and support (practical and emotional) of home care work is essential to better understand the reality of the care regimes. It is important that future comparative analysis studies do not neglect to focus on the delivery of services from the perspective of care workers and care recipients. This additional analysis could examine whether experiences and expectations differ across the sectors (that is, public, private and not-for-profit) and could help to elucidate whether an expansion of the care market serves to improve conditions for both care worker and care recipients. Whether observational methods should be used to conduct this analysis is open to debate. Where time permits, we would recommend the use of qualitative interviewing or a cross-country quantitative analysis, although the latter may be made difficult due to the fact that each questionnaire would have to be highly context specific.

Future studies may also attempt to focus on a number of issues which were beyond the confines of this research. For instance, this research investigated only the publicly funded domiciliary care systems within each of the three countries, and, hence, no consideration was given to privately funded care services. This omission is particularly noteworthy in the case of the United States, where private LTCI and private domiciliary care services are more important than the public programmes for the majority of older people who are not eligible for public social care services or benefits. There are also enormous disparities between the various state-plan personal care programmes and waiver programmes in the United States, and these differences received only cursory attention within this study.

The subject of informal care, of obvious relevance in the area of domiciliary care, was largely addressed from the perspective of policies and monetary recognition of informal caregivers. Reference was made to a number of studies carried out in the three countries on informal caregiving, but future research would clearly benefit from placing greater attention on the interface between formal and informal care, a crucial area that has received insufficient attention in the literature. Studies observing the interaction and respective roles of informal and formal caregivers would be particularly warranted as many domiciliary care policies apply to both, and as the ability to choose or alternate between these is of great relevance for the degree of consumer choice and direction.

Finally, the importance of complementing home care with voluntary ancillary community care supports was mentioned in interviews in Denmark, Germany and the United States and is something that could be examined in more detail in future research. Home care is care in the community and, as such, it can only blossom in communities where collectivism, unity and intergenerational (and intercultural) acceptance and appreciation flourish. It must also be realised that older people themselves are an important resource in discussions on future social care systems. Comparative research on domiciliary care has tended to focus on broader institutional frameworks – such a focus may not give sufficient attention to the specific needs of older people. A dialogue between policy makers and the chief beneficiaries of the domiciliary services must take place in order to discover where and how these care recipients want to be cared for, according to their various changing circumstances. Policy makers will succeed only when they genuinely engage with the current and future care recipients.

Bibliography

Abrahamson, P., T.P Boje and B. Greve (2005), *Welfare and Families in Europe*, Aldershot: Ashgate.

Alber, J. (1995), ‘A framework for the comparative study of social services’, *Journal of European Social Policy*, **5** (2), 131–49.

Anttonen, A. and J. Sipilä (1996), ‘European social care services: is it possible to identify models?’, *Journal of European Social Policy,* **6** (2), 87–100.

Aust, Andreas, Frank, Bönker, and Hellmut, Wollmann (2002), ‘Welfare state reform in Germany from 1982 to the present: Report for the 2002 WRAM-SOC conference, Kent.

Bahle, T. (2003), ‘The changing institutionalisation of social services in England and Wales, France and Germany: is the welfare state on the retreat?’, *Journal of European Social Policy*, **13** (1), 5–20.

Benjamin, A.E. and R.E. Matthias (2004), ‘Work-life differences and outcomes for agency and consumer-directed home-care workers’, *The Gerontologist,* **44** (4), 479–88.

Benjamin, A.E. and R.E. Matthias (2001), ‘Age, consumer direction, and outcomes of supportive services at home’, *The Gerontologist,* **41** (5), 632–42.

Benjamin, A.E. (2001), ‘Consumer-directed services at home: a new model for persons with disabilities’, *Health Affairs*, **20** (6), 80–96.

Benjamin, A.E., R.E. Matthias and T.M. Franke (1999) *Comparing Client-directed and Agency Models for Providing Supportive Services at Home,* report for the Assistant Secretary for Planning and Evaluation, HHS, US Department of Health and Human Services, April.

Benjamin, A.E., R.E. Matthias and T.M. Franke (2000), ‘Comparing consumer-directed and agency models for providing supportive services at home’, *Health Services Research*, **35**, 351–66.

Berkman, L. F. and T. Glass (2000) ‘Social integration, social networks, social support, and health’, (eds) L. F. Berkman and I. Kawachi in *Social Epidemiology*, New York: Oxford University Press, pp. 137–73.

Bönker, Frank and Hellmut Wollmann (2005), ‘Public sector reforms and local government in Germany: the case of local social policy’, forthcoming in Vincent Hoffmann-Martinot and Hellmut Wollmann (eds), *Comparing Public Sector Reforms in France and Germany*, Wiesbaden: VS.

Brodsky, Jenny, Jack Habib and Ilana Mizrahi (2000), *Long-term Care Laws in Five Developed Countries: A Review* (Publication no. WHO/NMH/CCL/00.2), Geneva: World Health Organization.

Bureau of Labor Statistics (2006), Occupational Employment Statistics May 2005, Washington, DC: US Bureau of Labor Statistics.

California Department of Social Services (2002), *IHSS: Keeping the Quality of Life at Home, In-Home Supportive Services Recipient Report*, CA: California Department of Social Services Data Analysis and Publication Branch.

Campbell, A.L. and K.J. Morgan (2005), 'Federalism and the politics of old-age care in Germany and the United States', *Comparative Political Studies*, **38** (8), 1–28.

Cox, Carole B. (2005), *Community Care for an Aging Society: Issues, Policies and Services*, New York: Springer.

Csonka, Agi and Joachim Lynggaard Boll (2001), 'Home care in Denmark'. in Emmanuel Mermet and Steffen Lehndorff (eds), *New Forms of Employment and Working Time in the Service Economy (NESY)*, Brussels: ETUI, pp. 233–41.

Cuellar A.E. and J.M. Wiener (2000), 'Can social insurance for long-term care work? The experience of Germany', *Health Affairs*, **19** (3), 8–25.

Cullen, Kevin, Sarah Delaney and Petrina Duff (2004), *Caring, Working and Public Policy*, Dublin: Equality Authority.

Daatland, S.O. and A. Lowenstein (2005), 'Intergenerational solidarity and the family-welfare state balance' *European Journal of Ageing*, **2** (3), 174–82.

Dallinger, Ursula (2002), 'Elderly care in the family in Germany' Paper presented at the European Cooperation in the field of Scientific and Technical Research (COST) 13A Meeting, Copenhagen, 19 April.

Daly, Donna, Jennifer Tucker-Tatlow and Carrie Gibson (2004), *In-Home Supportive Services: Characteristics, Cost Drivers and Cost Containment*, San Diego, CA: Southern Area Consortium of Human Services.

Daly, Mary (ed.) (2001), *Care Work: the Quest for Security. Geneva*, International Labour Organization.

Daly, Mary and Jane Lewis (1998), 'Introduction: conceptualising social care in the context of welfare state restructuring, in M. Daly and J. Lewis (eds), *Gender, Social Care and Welfare State Restructuring in Europ*e, Aldershot: Ashgate, pp. 1–24.

Danish Ministry of the Interior and Health (2004), *Agreement on a Structural Reform*, Copenhagen: Ministry of the Interior and Health.

Esping-Andersen, Gosta (1990), *The Three Worlds of Welfare Capitalism*, Cambridge: Polity.

Esping-Andersen, Gosta (1999), *Social Foundations of Postindustrial Economies*, Oxford: Oxford University Press.

European Commission (2003), *The Social Situation in the European Union 2003*, Luxembourg: EUR OP.

Evers, Adalbert (1995), 'The future of elderly care in Europe: limits and aspirations' in F. Scharf and C. Wenger (eds), *International Perspectives on Community Care for Older People*, Aldershot: Avebury, pp. 3–20.

Evers, Adalbert (1998), 'The new long-term care insurance program in Germany', *Journal of Aging and Social Policy*, **10**, 77–95.

Evers, Adalbert and Ivan Svetlik (eds) (1993), *Balancing Pluralism: New Welfare Mixes in Care for the Elderly*, Aldershot: Avebury.

Feder, J. (1999), 'Improving public financing for long-term care: the political challenge', *Journal of Aging and Social Policy*, **10** (3),1–6.

Feder, J., H.L. Komisar and M. Niefeld (2000), 'Long-term care in the United States: an overview', *Health Affairs*, **19** (3), 40–56.

Federal Ministry of Health and Social Security (2005) *Selected Facts and Figures about Long-term Care.* Ref-231\Unterlageden\Selected Facts and Figures, Bonn, April.

Ferrera, M. (1996), 'The southern model of welfare in social Europe', *Journal of European Social Policy*, **6** (1), 17–37.

Frade, Carlos and Isabelle Darmon (2005), 'New modes of business organization and precarious employment: towards the recommodification of labour?', *Journal of European Social Policy*, **15** (2), 107–21.

Freedman, V. (1996), 'Family structure and the risk of nursing home admission', *Journal of Gerontology: Social Sciences*, **51B** (2), 61–9.

Fries, J. (2003), 'Measuring and monitoring success in compressing morbidity', *Annals of Internal Medicine*, **139**, 455–9.

FOA (2005), 'Integration inden for social- og sundhedsområdet'. Forbundet af Offentligt Ansatte (FOA), Copenhagen.

Glendinning, Caroline and Gerhard Igl (forthcoming), 'Social policies for an ageing society: Britain and Germany compared', in Gerhard Naegele and Alan Walker (eds), *Social Policy in Ageing Societies: Britain and Germany Compared*, Basingstoke: Palgrave Macmillan.

Glendinning, C., B. Davies, L. Pickard and A. Comas-Herrera (2004), *Funding Long-term Care for Older People: Lessons from Other Countries*, Country Reports, York: Social Policy Research Unit and London: School of Economics, Personal Social Services Research Unit.

Green-Pedersen, Christoffer (2002), 'New public management reforms of the Danish and Swedish welfare states: the role of different social democratic responses', *Governance*, **15** (2), 271–94.

Groger, Lisa (2006), 'Gifts or poison? The cultural context of using public funds to pay family caregivers', in Suzanne Kunkel and Valerie Wellin (eds), *Consumer Voice and Choice in Long-term Care*, New York: Springer, pp. 221–32.

Grundy, Emily (2001), 'Ageing and vulnerable elderly people in Europe'. *Ageing, Intergenerational Solidarity, and Age-specific Vulnerability*, 20–21 April, Solicited Papers and Country Reports: Volume 1, Rome: Institute for Population Research, pp. 5–40.

Hendriksen C. and M. Vass (2005), 'Preventive home visits to elderly people in Denmark'. *Zeitschrift für Gerontologie und Geriatrie*, **38** (1), 31–3.

Hendriksen C., E. Lund and E. Stromgard (1984), 'Consequences of assessment and intervention among elderly people: a three-year randomized controlled trial', *British Medical Journal*, **289**, 1522–24.

Hirschman, Albert, O. (1970) *Exit, Voice, and Loyalty: Responses to Decline in Firms, Organizations, and States*, Cambridge, MA: Harvard University Press.

Holstein B.E, K. Avlund and R.L Heikkinen (1997), 'Home help and informal social support for elderly persons in three Nordic localities', *Facts, Research and Intervention in Geriatrics*, Supplement, 41–54.

Holstein, B.E., E.P Due, G. Almind and E. Holst (1991), 'The home-help service in Denmark', in A. Jamieson (ed.), *Home Care for Older People in Europe*, Oxford: Oxford University Press, pp. 38–62.

Howes, Candance (2005), 'The impact on worker income, health insurance coverage, and Medi-Cal CALWORKS and food stamp eligibility', Testimony before the California State Assembly Budget Committee Hearings on Proposed Cuts in State Match to IHSS Wage and Benefit Costs, 6 April.

Jacobzone, S. (2000), 'Health and ageing: international perspectives on long-term care', *Isuma Canadian Journal of Policy Research*, **1** (2) www.isuma.net/v01n02/jacobzone/-jacobzone_e.shtml [19 June, 2007].

Jarden, M.E. and J.O. Jarden (2002), 'Social and health-care policy for the elderly in Denmark', Global Action on Aging, www.globalaging.org/elderrights/world/-densocialhealthcare.htm [19 June, 2007].

Jensen, Jytte Juul and Helle Krogh Hansen (2002), 'Mapping of care services and the care workforce in Denmark', *Care Work in Europe: Current Understandings and Future Directions*, Forskningsrapport 78 sider, www.carework.dk, [19 June, 2007].

Kane R.L., R.A. Kane, R.C. Ladd and W.N. Veazie (1998), 'Variation in state spending for long-term care: factors associated with more balanced systems'. *Journal of Health Politics, Policy and Law*, **23** (2), 363–90.

Karlsson, Martin, Les Mayhew, Robert Plumb and Ben Rickayzen (2004), 'An international comparison of long-term care arrangements. An investigation into the equity, efficiency and sustainability of the long-term care systems in Germany, Japan, the United Kingdom and the United States', Actuarial Research Paper No. 156, Actuarial Research Centre, Cass Business School, London.

Kautto, M. (2002), 'Investing in services in West European welfare states', *Journal of European Social Policy,* **12** (1), 53–65.

Kitchener, M. and C. Harrington (2004), 'The U.S long-term care field: a dialectic analysis of institution dynamics', *Journal of Health and Social Behavior*, 45 (extra issue), p. 87–101.

Kitchener, M., T. Ng and C. Harrington (2004), 'Medicaid 1915(c) home and community-based services waivers: a national survey of eligibility criteria, caps, and waiting lists', *Home Health Care Services Quarterly*, **23** (2), 55–69.

Kitchener, M., T. Ng and C. Harrington (2002), 'Medicaid Home and Community-Based Services Data', Center for Personal Assistance Services, San Francisco: University of California, San Francisco, http://pascenter.org/medicaid/ [19 June, 2007].

Kohl, J. (1981), 'Trends and problems in public expenditure development in Western Europe and North America', in P. Flora and Arnold Heidenheimer (eds), *The Development of Welfare States in Europe and America*, London: Transaction Books, pp. 307–46.

Korczyk, Sophie (2004), *Long-term Workers in Five Countries: Issues and Options,* Washington, DC: AARP Public Policy Institute.

Kröger, Teppo (2001), *Comparative Research on Social Care: The State of the Art*, Brussels: European Commission.

Lethbridge, Jane (2005), 'Changing care policies in Europe', Background paper for workshop held in Budapest on Social Services and Social Dialogue in Europe, organised by EPSU and ETUCO 17–20 March 2005, Published 24 February 2005, London: Public Services International Research Unit (PSIRU).

Lewinter, Myra (2004), 'Developments in home help for elderly people in Denmark: the changing concept of home and institution', *International Journal of Social Welfare*, **13** (1) 89–96.

Lewis, Jane (2000), 'Gender and welfare regimes', in Gail Lewis, Sharon Gewirtz and John Clarke (eds), *Rethinking Social Policy,* London: Sage, pp. 37–51.

Lundsgaard, Jens (2005), 'Consumer direction and choice in long-term care for older persons, including payments for informal care: how can it help improve care outcomes, employment and fiscal sustainability?', OECD Health Working Paper No. 20, Paris: OECD.

Mayer, K.U. and M. Wagner (1996), 'Lebenslage und soziale Ungleicheit im hohen Alter', in K.U Mayer and P.B. Balter (eds), *Die Berliner Alterss-tudie*, Berlin: Akademie Verlag, pp. 251–75.

Meijer, A., C. van Campen and A. Kerskta (2000), 'A comparative study of the financing, provision and quality of care in nursing homes. The approach of four European countries: Belgium, Denmark, Germany and the Netherlands', *Journal of Advanced Nursing*, **32** (3), 554–61.

Merlis, M. (2000), 'Caring for the frail elderly: an international review', *Health Affairs,* **5** (6), 141–49.

Ministry of Social Affairs (2002), *Social Policy in Denmark*, Copenhagen: Ministry of Social Affairs.

Morel, Nathalie (2006), 'From subsidiarity to "free choice": child- and elderly-care policy reforms in France, Germany, Belgium and the Netherlands', Paper prepared for the workshop: A long goodbye to Bismark? The politics of welfare reforms in Continental Europe, organized by Bruno Palier and Peter A. Hall at the Center for European Studies, Harvard University, 16–17 June.

O'Brien, Martin and Sue Penna (1998), *Theorising Welfare: Enlightenment and Modern Society,* London: Sage.

OECD (2005), *The OECD Health Project: Long-term Care for Older People*, Paris: OECD.

OECD (2006), *OECD Health Data 2006*, Paris: OECD.

Pacolet, Jozef (2001), 'Social protection and ageing in Europe: a supply side approach', *Ageing, Intergenerational Solidarity, and Age-specific Vulnerability,* 20–21 April, Solicited Papers and Country Reports: Volume 1, Rome: Institute for Population Research, pp. 41–76.

Paraprofessional Healthcare Institute (2006), 'Who are direct care workers?,' National Clearinghouse on Direct Care Workforce Fact Sheet, New York: November.

Pierce, Maria (2006), 'Older people and social care', in Bryan Fanning and Michael Rush (eds), *Care and Social Change in the Irish Welfare Economy*, Dublin: University College Dublin Press, pp. 190–205.

Rostgaard, Tine (2004), 'The construction of consumerism – free choice of care for the elderly in Denmark', Paper presented at the Symposium on Consumerism of Care for the Elderly organized by the Danish National Institute of Social Research (SFI), Copenhagen, 30 August.

Rostgaard, Tine and Torben Fridberg (1998), *Caring for Children and Older People: A Comparison of European Policies and Practices,* Copenhagen: Danish National Institute of Research.

Rothgang, Heinz (2003), 'Long-term care for older people in Germany', in Adelina Comas-Herrera and Raphael Wittenberg (eds), *European Study of Long Term Expenditure*, Report to the European Commission, Employment and Social Affairs DG, PSSRU, Discussion Paper 1840, Brussels.

Samuelsson, Gills (2000), 'The quality of home care services in Sweden consumer: expectations and changing satisfaction', in Anthony M. Warnes, Lorna Warnen and Michael Nolan (eds), *Care Services for Later Life: Transformations and Critiques,* London: Jessica Kingsley, pp. 184–203.

Sarantakos, Sotirios (2005), *Social Research* (3rd ed.), Basingstoke: Palgrave Macmillan.

Scharf, Thomas and Clare Wenger (1995), 'International perspectives on community care,' in T. Scharf and C. Wenger (eds) *International Perspectives on Community Care for Older People*, Aldershot: Avebury, pp. 217–20.

Scharlach, A., K. Gustavson and T. Dal Santo (forthcoming), 'Assistance received by employed caregivers and their care recipients: who helps care recipients when caregivers work full-time?', *The Gerontologist.*

Scharlach, A., B. Sirotnik, S. Bockman, M. Neiman, C. Ruiz and T. Dal Santo, (2003), 'A profile of family caregivers: results of the California Statewide Survey of Caregivers', San Francisco: University of California at Berkeley, Center for the Advanced Study of Aging Services, School of Social Welfare.

Scharlach, A., T. Dal Santo, A. Lehning, K. Gustavson, S. Lee, E. Auh, P. Fox and J. Chow (2006), 'Caregiving in California: final report of the University of California Family Caregiver Support Project', San Francisco: University of California at Berkeley, Center for the Advanced Study of Aging Services, School of Social Welfare.

Schneeklooth, U. and U. Müller (2000), *Wirkungen der Pflegeversicherung*, Baden-Baden: Nomas.

Schultz-Larsen, K., S. Kreiner, S. Hanning, N. Støvring, K.D. Hansen and S. Lendal (2004), *The Danish Eldercare under Change: A Controlled, Randomised Intervention Study of Eldercare in 36 Municipalities*, Copenhagen: The Institute of Public Health, University of Copenhagen, in cooperation with the Centre for Research and Development in Eldercare.

Sciegaj, M., J.A. Capitman and K. Kyriacou (2004), 'Consumer-directed community care: race/ethnicity and individual differences in preferences for control', *The Gerontologist*, **44** (4), 489–99.

Sjørup, Karen (2004), 'The Danish care for the elderly in a gender mainstreaming perspective', Paper presented at the Gender Analysis and Long-term Care Assistance conference, Economic and Social Research Institute, Dublin, 30 April.

Stack, S. and C. Provis (2000), 'Tensions in flexible employment arrangements for caring labour', Proceedings of 14th AIRAANZ Conference (Newcastle, February), ed. J. Burgess and G. Strachan, vol. 2, pp. 162–171.

StBA (Statistisches Bundesamt) (2001), *Kurzbericht Pflegestatistik 1999 – Pflege im Rahmen der Pfegeversicherung – Deutschlandergebnisse,* Wiesbaden: Statistisches Bundesamt.

Stone, R. (2001), 'Providing long-term care benefits in cash: moving to a disability model', *Health Affairs*, **20** (6), 96–108.

Stone, R. (2004), 'The direct care worker: a key dimension of home care policy', *Home Health Care Management and Practice*, **16** (5), 339–49.

Stuart, M. and M. Weinrich (2001), 'Home- and community-based long-term care: lessons from Denmark', *The Gerontologist,* **41** (4) 474–80.

Stuck, A., M. Egger, A. Hammer, C.E. Minder and J.C. Beck (2002), 'Home visits to prevent nursing home admission and functional decline in elderly people. Systematic review and meta-analysis', *Journal of the American Medical Association*, **287**,1022–8.

Tester, Susan (1996), *Community Care for Older People: A Comparative Perspective*. Basingstoke: Macmillan.

Theobald, Hildegard (2003), 'Care for the elderly: welfare system, professionalisation and the question of inequality', in B. Blättel-Mink and E. Kuhlmann (eds), *Health Professions, Gender and Society: Shifting Relations in Times of Institutional and Social Change, International Journal of Sociology and Social Policy,* Special Issue, **23** (4/5), 159–85.

Theobald, Hildegard (2005), 'Evaluation of results of care arrangement study under consideration of a comparative perspective on the impact of welfare states on marginalization of the aged', Unpublished report EU-Project: Care for the Aged at Risk of Marginalization (CARMA).

Timonen, Virpi (2005), 'Policy paradigms and long-term care: convergence or continuing difference', in Peter Taylor-Gooby (ed.) *Ideas and Welfare State Reform in Western Europe*, Basingstoke: Palgrave Macmillan, pp. 30–53.

Timonen Virpi, Martha Doyle and David Prendergast (2006), *No Place Like Home: Study of Domiciliary Care Services for Older People in Ireland*, Dublin: Liffey Press.

Titmuss, Richard M. (1974), *Social Policy: An Introduction*, London: Allen & Unwin.

Twigg, Julia (2000), *Bathing: The Body and Community Care*, London: Routledge.

US Census (2005), http://quickfacts.census.gov/qfd/states/00000.html [19 June, 2007].

US Department of Health and Human Services (2000), *Understanding Medicaid Home and Community Services: A Primer*, Washington, DC: U.S. Department of Health and Human Services, Office of the Assistant Secretary for Planning and Evaluation.

United Nations Population Division (2000), *World Population Prospects: The 2000 Revision*, New York: United Nations.

Ungerson, C. (2004), 'Whose empowerment and independence? A cross-national perspective on "cash for care" schemes', *Ageing and Society*, **24** (2), 189–212.

Vallgårda, Signild, Allan Krasnik and Karsten Vrangbæk (2001), *Health Care Systems in Transition: Denmark,* European Observatory on Health Care Systems, Copenhagen: WHO.

Wellin, Chris (2006), 'Scrutinizing familial care in consumer-directed long-term care programmes: implications for theory and research', in Suzanne

Kunkel and Valerie Wellin (eds), *Consumer Voice and Choice in Long-term Care*, New York: Springer, pp. 195–220.

Wiener, J.M. and A.E Cuellar (1999), 'Public and private responsibilities: home- and community-based services in the United Kingdom and Germany', *Journal of Aging and Health*, **11** (3), 417–44.

Wiener, J.M. and D.G. Stevenson (1998), 'State Policy on long-term care for the elderly', *Health Affairs*, **17** (3), 81–100.

World Health Organization (WHO) (2002), *Current and Future Long-term Care Needs: An Analysis Based on the 1990 WHO Study: The Global Burden of Disease*, Geneva: WHO.

Index